Examination Preparation

A Complete Guide for the Physical Therapist

Scott M. Giles M.S., P.T.

Clinical Assistant Professor
Department of Physical Therapy
University of New England
Biddeford, Maine

Ronda Sanders M.Ed, CET

Assistant Professor
Department of Learning Assistance and Individual Learning
University of New England
Biddeford, Maine

Mainely Physical Therapy
P.O. Box 7242
Scarborough, Maine 04070-7242

Phone: (207) 885-0304
Fax: (207) 883-8377
Website: www.ptexams.com
email: ptexams@cybertours.com

ACKNOWLEDGMENTS

We would like to offer our sincere thanks
to Therese Giles and Dr. Jaime Hylton
for their valuable assistance
with this project.

CONTENTS

Introduction

Unit Seven   Final Preparation

Unit Eight   Sample Examination

Bibliography

Appendix

Activity Log
Time Management Diagnostic Sheet
Relaxation Exercise
Resource List
Order Forms

Introduction

The word examination can strike fear and anxiety into individuals like few other words in the English language. What is it about an examination that is so threatening to the majority of the population? The American Heritage Dictionary defines the word examination as "a set of questions designed to test knowledge." Although students are frequently exposed to examinations throughout their academic training, the thought of a comprehensive examination can make even the sturdiest student begin to perspire.

In physical therapy, the ultimate comprehensive examination is the Physical Therapist Examination. The national examination serves to measure the knowledge and skills necessary for minimal competency in the field of physical therapy and is often the final hurdle a physical therapist must clear before obtaining licensure.

Perhaps a candidate's apprehension can be more clearly understood when viewing the significance of this examination. Candidates, in most cases, have recently completed their academic preparation and are eager to embark on their professional careers. They recognize that failure to meet or exceed the minimum scoring requirement on the examination can act as a barrier prohibiting them from practicing as an independent professional.

Our text is designed to maximize a candidate's performance on the Physical Therapist Examination. The text will accomplish this goal by taking candidates through eight distinct and separate units.

Unit One - Physical Therapist Examination

Unit One provides in depth information on the Physical Therapist Examination. It outlines the purpose, format and design of the examination and addresses issues ranging from registration to scoring.

Unit Two - Time Management

Unit Two allows candidates to assess their time management skills. Candidates are presented with useful guidelines to consider when designing a study schedule.

Unit Three - You as a Learner

Unit Three provides candidates with the opportunity to assess their individual learning style. Candidates are shown how this information can be utilized as they prepare for the Physical Therapist Examination.

Unit Four - Study Plan

Unit Four explores the many different components of an effective study plan. Candidates are presented with valuable information to guide them as they develop an individualized study plan.

Unit Five - Multiple Choice Examinations

Unit Five analyzes the various components of a multiple choice examination. Suggested techniques to assist candidates when analyzing a multiple choice question are introduced. Candidates are given the opportunity to refine their test taking skills by answering selected examination questions.

Unit Six - Content Outline

Unit Six provides candidates with the opportunity to explore the content outline of the Physical Therapist Examination. A summary of each of the categories within the content outline is provided along with selected sample questions.

Unit Seven - Final Preparation

Unit Seven discusses issues for candidates to consider on the final days prior to the Physical Therapist Examination. Specific strategies to maximize performance and limit anxiety are discussed.

Unit Eight - Sample Examination

Unit Eight consists of a sample 200 question examination. Candidates are given the opportunity to refine their test taking skills and to assess their level of preparedness for the actual examination.

Unit One
Physical Therapist Examination

The Physical Therapist Examination is a 200 question, multiple choice examination. The examination is designed to determine if candidates possess the minimal competency necessary to practice as physical therapists.

The examination is created under the auspices of the Federation of State Boards of Physical Therapy. According to the <u>Examination Handbook for Physical Therapist and Physical Therapist Assistant</u>, the national examination program serves two important purposes:

1. provide examination services to regulatory boards charged with the licensing of physical therapists and physical therapist assistants.

2. provide a common element in evaluation of candidates so that standards will be comparable from state/jurisdiction to state/jurisdiction.

Registration

Registration occurs at the state level through the Physical Therapy State Licensing Agencies. The address of each agency and a corresponding phone number are provided in the Appendix. Many of the state licensing agencies have very different eligibility requirements; therefore it is imperative that all application forms are read carefully.

A variety of items may be required as part of the application process. These items include a photograph; a notarized birth certificate; an official transcript from an accredited school; professional reference letters; and a check or money order for the required application, examination, and licensing fees.

It can not be emphasized enough, however, that individual state licensing agencies' requirements vary. One small example is that many states will not accept any form of payment other than a money order or a certified bank check. If an applicant uses another form of payment, such as a personal check, the application could be considered incomplete. To avoid such difficulties, it is prudent to read the application carefully and to inquire as to the status of the application approximately two weeks after the completed application has been submitted.

Some states offer candidates the opportunity to practice prior to being licensed by issuing a temporary permit. Typically, candidates are required to have a completed application on file and have met all other qualifications for licensure before being considered for the permit. Temporary permits are usually revoked if a candidate receives notification he/she was not successful on the Physical Therapist Examination.

Licensure

There are two primary ways in which to obtain a license to practice as a physical therapist. They are termed examination and endorsement.

Examination

Licensure by examination is obtained after a candidate meets or exceeds the minimum scoring requirement on the Physical Therapist Examination and has satisfied all other state requirements. This form of obtaining licensure is the traditional method for candidates seeking initial licensure.

Endorsement

Licensure by endorsement makes it possible for candidates who have been licensed in a state by virtue of an examination to potentially gain licensure in another state without retaking the examination. Examination scores can be transferred to any physical therapy state licensing agency via the Interstate Reporting Service of Professional Examination Service. The address of the Interstate Reporting Service is available in the Appendix.

Foreign Trained Therapists

Foreign trained therapists often are subjected to a myriad of requirements before they are eligible to become licensed in the United States. Since the requirements vary significantly by state, it is recommended that candidates contact the physical therapy state licensing agency within the state they intend to practice. The state licensing agency can then provide detailed information on their individual requirements.

There are two general requirements which seem to be consistent in all states for foreign trained therapists:

1. Applicants are required to submit their educational credentials for evaluation of their equivalence to the United States trained applicant.

2. Applicants must meet or exceed the minimum scoring requirement on the Physical Therapist Examination.

Other state requirements can include, but are not limited to, the following:

- demonstrate proficiency in written and spoken English
- submit letters of reference
- obtain a valid visa and resident alien card
- complete an internship or period of supervised practice
- appear for an interview
- attain the equivalent of a United States grade of "C" or higher in all professional coursework

Examination Development

According to the Federation of State Boards of Physical Therapy, the Physical Therapist Examination is developed by three committees. These committees are the Examination Construction and Review Committee; the Item Bank Review Committee; and the Item Writer and Review Committee.

The Examination Construction and Review Committee is responsible for determining the content categories of the examination and the percentage of items in each category. The categories are based on the tasks and roles that comprise the practice of physical therapy. The information necessary to create each category is obtained after analyzing the responses of several hundred therapists to a job analysis survey.

Individual physical therapists have direct involvement in the writing of examination questions. The physical therapists involved are required to attend item-writing workshops that are taught by experienced testing professionals. Questions, once completed, are analyzed independently to make sure they are reflective of the current examination content outline. The focus of the examination questions is on problem solving and away from rote memorization of fact. Candidates are required to demonstrate their ability to apply knowledge in a safe and effective manner within a clinical setting.

Examination Administration

In 1999 computer based testing became the only mode of administration for the Physical Therapist Examination. Candidates begin the application process by obtaining a general application form and a computerized scannable information form from a participating state licensing agency. Once completed, the forms are returned along with any necessary fees to the state licensing agency. After a candidate's application is approved, the state licensing agency forwards the computerized form to Professional Examination Service.

Professional Examination Service scans the computerized form and sends the candidate information on how to schedule to take the examination. Candidates must sit for the examination within 60 days of the date on the eligibility letter from Professional Examination Service.

Candidates can take the examination at any of the 250 Sylvan Technology Centers within the United States or at selected testing facilities in Canada. Testing is offered Monday through Saturday from 9:00 AM - 6:00 PM. Within each Sylvan Technology Center candidates can concentrate on the examination without environmental distracters. Private, modular booths provide adequate work space with proper lighting and ventilation. All Sylvan Technology Centers are fully accessible.

Candidates are not limited to the testing centers within the state they are applying for licensure. For example, a student that has recently graduated from a physical therapy program in Maine could apply for licensure in California and take the required examination while still in Maine.

It is important to note that basic computer skills are not necessary with computer based testing. Prior to beginning the examination, candidates utilize a tutorial which explains topics such as selecting answers and navigating within the examination. Time spent on the computer tutorial does not count towards the allotted time for the actual examination.

Candidates are given the option of entering their answers using a computer keyboard or mouse. Once within the actual examination candidates can move freely between examination questions. Candidates can go back to previously answered or unanswered questions and make any desired changes. Candidates are allowed to use scratch paper supplied by the testing center during the examination.

Content Outline

The content outline provides candidates with a detailed description of the information contained on the Physical Therapist Examination. Although listed here, the content outline will be discussed in detail in Unit Six.

Physical Therapist Examination

I. Assessment and Evaluation

    A. General Procedures
        1. Data Collection
        2. Test/Measurements
    B. System Specific Procedures

II. Interpretation and Planning

    A. Data Interpretation
    B. Goal Setting and Care Planning

III. Intervention

    A. Preparation
    B. Implementation
    C. Education/Communication/Consultation
    D. Supporting Activities
    E. System Specific Procedures

Scoring

In July of 2000, 25 pretest items were added to each 200 question examination. This action allows pretest items to be evaluated throughout the year and eliminates lengthy delays in score reporting in July and August. Candidates are unable to differentiate between pretest and scored items on the 225 question examination. To accomodate for the increased number of questions, candidates receive an additional 30 minutes to complete the examination. Candidates have a total of 4.5 hours to complete the 225 question examination. Since candidate performance is based solely on the number of scored items answered correctly, the sample examination in Unit Eight consists of 200 questions.

An independent testing firm, Professional Examination Service, is responsible for scoring the examination and reporting results to the individual state licensing agencies. The state licensing agencies then send written notification to candidates as to their performance on the examination.

The questions are multiple choice with four possible answers to each question. Candidates are asked to identify the best answer to each of the questions. Each question has only one correct answer. A candidate's score is determined based on the number of questions answered correctly. Candidates accumulate one point for each correctly answered question. There is no penalty for questions answered incorrectly. The total cumulative score is termed the total raw score. The maximum total raw score for the Physical Therapist Examination is 200.

Criterion-referenced scoring is used to determine passing scores on the National Physical Therapy Examinations. Passing scores are determined based on the judgment of selected experts on the minimum number of questions that should be answered correctly by a minimally qualified candidate. Criterion-referenced passing scores are determined independently of candidate performance and are designed to reflect the difficulty of each examination. For example, if a given examination was judged to be particularly difficult, the minimum passing score would be lower than another examination that was judged to be less difficult.

Since the minimum passing score is based on the difficulty of the examination, it becomes impossible to determine an automatic passing score. Typically criterion-referenced passing scores range from 145 - 155. If the criterion-referenced passing score was established as 152 for a given examination, a total raw score of greater than or equal to 152 would be considered a passing score, while a total raw score of less than 152 would be considered a failing score.

An individual examination score is often reported to candidates in the form of a scaled score. Scaled scores range from 200 - 800 with the minimum passing score always being equal to a scaled score of 600.

If a candidate successfully completes the examination, in most cases he/she has fulfilled the final requirements for licensure. Conversely, if a candidate is unsuccessful on the examination, he/she is required to reapply to the state licensing agency. With computer based testing there is no mandatory waiting period before retaking the examination, however some states limit the number of times a candidate can take the examination or mandate remedial coursework in the event of multiple failures.

Candidates that were unsuccessful on the Physical Therapist Examination can elect to receive role feedback. The role feedback report compares individual examination performance with that of other candidates that took the same examination. Additional information on role feedback is available through Professional Examination Service.

Coming Attractions

As you have progressed through this unit, you most likely have gained an appreciation for the complexity of preparing for the Physical Therapist Examination. Although this task can, at times, seem overwhelming, there are a number of strategies that can significantly enhance a candidate's preparation efficiency and organization. These areas are:

- Time management skills
- A viable study plan
- Knowledge of how you learn
- Test taking skills

Each of these four areas will be discussed in detail in upcoming units. Candidates should attempt to apply the information obtained in these units as they prepare for the Physical Therapist Examination.

Unit Two
Time Management

Time management is, perhaps, the most overlooked component of a comprehensive study plan. Most candidates take the Physical Therapist Examination shortly after graduation. This can be a very anxious and unsettled time. Candidates often are actively seeking employment or are attempting to adjust to a new job. They may have relocated to a different residence or perhaps moved to another part of the country. To further complicate matters, they are starting to focus on the impending Physical Therapist Examination.

Time Management Assessment

Time management is not about meeting deadlines and getting things done. Time management is about keeping our lives in balance. We will classify the major areas of our lives into four distinct and separate categories. These areas are listed and defined below:

The emotional you:	your inner self - your ongoing and ever-changing perceptions and reflections on life, self, values, etc.
The intellectual you:	your intellectually curious self - student, reader, researcher, newswatcher, etc.
The physical you:	your physical self - walking, running, swimming, grooming, etc.
The social you:	your outer self - social interactions with family, friends, church activities, etc.

When the balance among these four areas is disturbed, stress inevitably results. One of the major by-products of stress is the inability to concentrate and retain information. Failure to concentrate while preparing for a comprehensive examination such as the Physical Therapist Examination can have devastating results.

How balanced are your days? Find out by keeping an Activity Log for a three day period. A sample Activity Log is located in the Appendix. Attempt to follow your normal daily routine during these three days. At the end of each day, summarize your activity using the Time Management Diagnostic Sheet.

TIME MANAGEMENT DIAGNOSTIC SHEET

	Day One	Day Two	Day Three	Total
CLASS				
STUDY				
INDIVIDUAL TIME				
SOCIAL TIME				
EXERCISE				
WORK				
SLEEP				
NAP				
NIGHT				
SPECIAL APPOINTMENTS				

After completing the diagnostic activity sheet, attempt to determine how balanced your days are. Ask yourself if there are any of the four areas of your life that are not represented in your daily activities. If deficient areas are identified, attempt to select activities to augment these areas.

Are you getting some physical activity? A twenty minute walk may be **sufficient**. Did you find time, or did you simply not get around to it? Was it too cold out, or **did you** simply not feel like exercising?

How about your social self? These times would include social functions, conversations with friends and family, or non-working lunches. Did you avoid others because you were not feeling very sociable, or did you feel you had too much to do without wasting time "playing?"

Did you nurture your emotional self? This reflective area of life is the most diverse among people, and often the most neglected. Some people serve their emotional needs in church, some like to meditate or listen to music. Did you avoid such activities because you felt you simply did not have the time to spare or did you feel it was relatively unimportant with all of your other pressing needs?

How about intellectual stimulation? Probably at this point your intellectual self is being pandered to for many hours each day preparing for the examination. However, it is healthy to have a few other intellectual pursuits not related to the examination. Have you placed other intellectual pursuits like reading the newspaper or watching the news on hold because you are immersed in preparing for the examination with every waking moment?

Candidates also need to assess their ability to concentrate. Do you find yourself drifting off and glancing at the clock to discover that twenty minutes have elapsed and you have no idea where the time went? Do you feel that your study breaks seem to get longer as your study session progresses? Do you elect not to take study breaks and find yourself waking up in the cold, early hours of the morning, slumped over your books with a sore neck? Can you find a million "necessary" chores to do in order to avoid settling down to study?

If you answered yes to any of the preceding questions, you may benefit from improved time management. Remember, stress is progressive, so the ability to concentrate and retain information will decrease as time goes on. We suggest that you try the following two-part program:

Time Management Program

Part One   Long-Range Planning

    Step 1:   Find a calendar and identify the months between now and the examination.

    Step 2:   Use the content outline and begin to assign time to each of the three content areas. Dedicate some available time to each of the three content areas so that they can be reviewed adequately prior to the examination.

           Since the three content areas vary significantly in their weighting, it is imperative that candidates also weight the study time dedicated to each area. The specific weighting of each of the content areas is discussed in detail in Unit Six.

           A sample three-month, long-range schedule is illustrated on the next page.

SAMPLE THREE MONTH LONG RANGE SCHEDULE

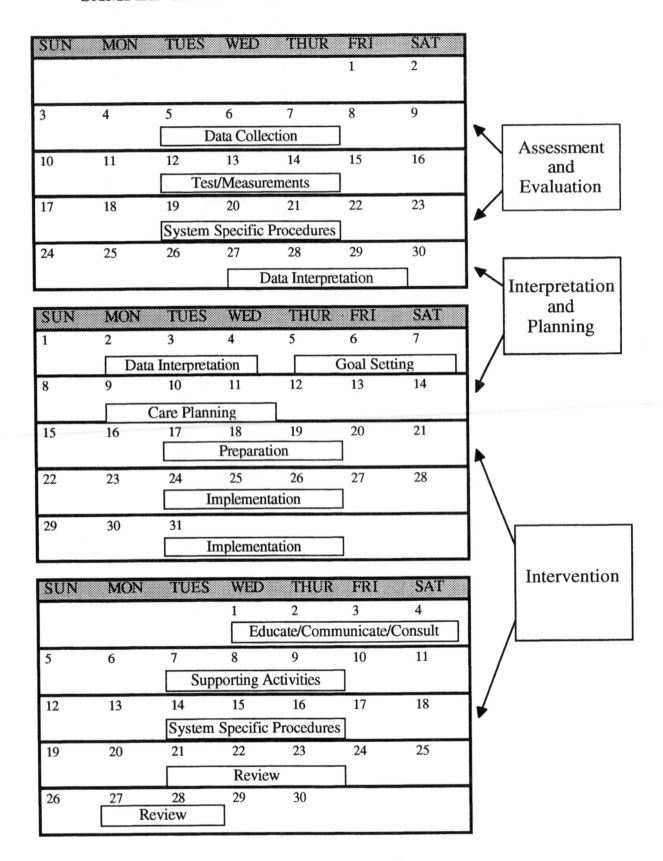

Part Two   Weekly Planning

Step 1:   Assign a color to each of the four areas of your life: emotional, intellectual, physical, and social.

Step 2:   Develop a master weekly schedule that includes all of your scheduled activities. These activities can include items such as: study sessions, work, church, social engagements and exercise sessions. Mark each of the activities that appear on the master schedule with the appropriate color.

Step 3:   Determine which, if any, of the four areas is being neglected in your present schedule. Select activities that can augment the deficient areas and assign them times, keeping in mind the following:

Emotional: individual reflection time allocated for thinking about issues important to you; done independently, goal-directed, resolution- oriented, time-limited; most people plan for one half-hour or two-fifteen minute periods daily, neither just before bed.

Intellectual: involves study time or clinical practice; follow the study plan suggested for your learning style, taking into consideration your learning environment preferences (Unit Three).

Physical: works best if not done immediately after a meal or just before bedtime; combines well with emotional or social time immediately afterwards.

Social: includes meal time, movies, theater, etc; works best when scheduled before a firm commitment, since individuals are most likely to lose track of time in this area.

Step 4:   Complete the schedule, being sure to leave at least one hour each day unfilled. When a scheduled activity is missed, it can be rescheduled easily within the available time.

Step 5:   Follow the schedule for at least one week and then do a self-assessment of your satisfaction with your productivity and concentration during study times. You may find it necessary to make adjustments to your future schedule based on your progress or lack thereof.

The following table illustrates a sample weekly schedule, which has been coded to correspond to each of the four areas of your life. By quickly examining the schedule, it becomes fairly easy to determine the relative weighting of each area. Candidates should attempt to design an individual schedule that is consistent with their present life status.

SAMPLE WEEKLY TIME MANAGEMENT SCHEDULE

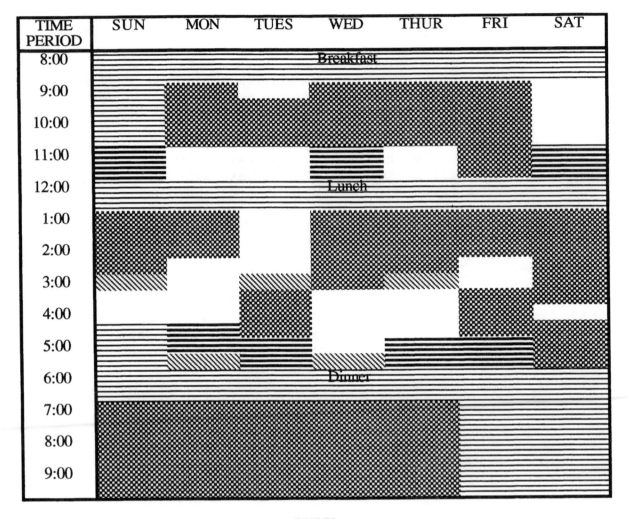

KEY

Emotional		Intellectual	
Physical		Social	
	Free Time		

Unit Three
You as a Learner

We imagine that at some time during your college years, you have observed the most obnoxious learner of all, the one who never seems to study and then consistently receives an "A" on every examination. This person does not necessarily have any more intelligence than other students, but simply may have developed a sense of how he/she learns most efficiently and is therefore able to develop a study plan based on his/her individual learning needs. It is our hope that the time management strategies presented earlier, in combination with the material that will be conveyed in this unit, will enable you to develop an efficient and effective individualized study plan.

To discover how you function as a learner, you need to answer three specific questions:

1. What combination of the three learning channels do you prefer for input and processing?
2. What is your dominant thinking mode?
3. What is your optimum learning environment?

The Three Learning Channels

There are three basic ways of perceiving information: see it (visual), hear it (auditory), or be physically involved in doing it (tactile/kinesthetic). The combination of these channels that an individual uses, both the first time he/she is exposed to new material (input) and during subsequent exposure (processing), determines one of the facets of learning style. Each individual's preference of channels for input and processing determines Active/Passive learning patterns.

Attempt to classify your preferred learning style for input and processing into one of the following four categories:

Active/Active

If you are an individual who, the first time you are exposed to new material likes to hear it, see it, say it, question it, interact with it, and then keep right on doing this, you would be categorized as a multisensoral (visual, auditory, and tactile/kinesthetic) active learner for both input and processing. These individuals immediately attempt to determine the relevance and utility of material and must, at input, be able to relate it to previous knowledge or experience. They typically find it difficult, and sometimes impossible, to go into a room alone, open up a book, and read.

Strengths:

- focus on application and utility of ideas
- 100% concentration on activities for short periods of time
- flexibility and adaptability

15

Weaknesses:

- may consider details boring
- short attention span may lead to incomplete preparation
- high distractibility may disrupt concentration

Active/Passive

If you are an individual who, the first time you are exposed to new material, likes to hear it, see it, say it, question it, interact with it, and then take a visual reference home to study by yourself, you would be classified as multisensoral learner for input and a visual processor. These individuals need to relate new material, at input, to previous knowledge or experience.

Strengths:

- focus on gathering extensive data
- long term memory
- strong visual channel often allows them to visualize notes, text, charts in their mind's eye

Weaknesses:

- may not focus on utility or use of information
- may require more time to learn new material
- may have a tendency to gather excessive information in an area of special interest and neglect other important areas

Passive/Active

If you are an individual who, the first time you are exposed to new material, likes either to hear it in lecture form or to read it in a book, and then utilize the material in an interactive way (visual, auditory, tactile/kinesthetic), you would be categorized as a passive learner for input and an active processor. These individuals relate new material to previous knowledge or experience and determine the relevance and utility of the material after input and before processing.

Strengths:

- focus on both facts/concepts and clinical application
- synthesis of known information into a plan of action
- sequential and relational thought

Weaknesses:

- may have difficulty determining proportional importance of information
- may begin applying information before sufficient details have been gathered
- may fail to identify the relationship to previous knowledge or experience

Passive/Passive

If you are an individual who, the first time you are exposed to new material, likes either to hear it or to read it and prefers to keep right on doing that, you would be categorized as a passive learner for both input and processing. These individuals determine the relationship to known material after input and before processing.

Strengths:

- sequential thinking
- focus on details
- strong visual channel that allows one to visualize notes, text, charts in their mind's eye

Weaknesses:

- may miss the "big picture"
- may have difficulty answering application questions requiring relational thinking
- tendency to study alone often inhibits opportunities to examine information from different perspectives

Once you have identified your preferred learning style for input and processing, attempt to classify the strength of your preference. We have divided this category into slight, decided and strong.

If all of the descriptors in one of the categories describe your learning style, place a check under strong preference. If the majority, but not all of the descriptors were accurate, place a check next to decided. If a few more of the descriptors in one category, when compared to the others, describe your learning style, place a check next to slight.

The stronger one's preference for a specific category, the less flexible a candidate will be in his/her input and processing channel needs. Candidates with a strong preference will need to pay particular attention to the recommendations for their learning style in Unit Four.

Input/Processing Preferences			
	Slight	Decided	Strong
Active/Active	☐	☐	☐
Active/Passive	☐	☐	☐
Passive/Active	☐	☐	☐
Passive/Passive	☐	☐	☐

Thinking Modes

You probably have heard the terms "left-brained" and "right-brained." In this book, these are not physiological or psychological terms, but instead educational terms which describe a set of learning characteristics. The following table depicts "left-brain" and "right-brain" learners' characteristics:

"Left" Thinking	"Right" Thinking
Facts	"What if.....?"
Words	Pictures
Sequences	Relationships
Details	Global concepts
Analytical	Synthetic

Complete the following informal exercise to evaluate your thinking mode.

1. Look over the text and the chart. Both contain the same information. Assume you are attempting to learn the information for the first time and that you have no previous knowledge of fruits' shape or color.

> **Fruits come in many shapes and colors. Oranges, kiwi, and tangerines are round; bananas are oblong; and pears are "pear shaped."**
>
> **Oranges and tangerines are orange; bananas and pears are yellow; kiwi is green.**

	Shape			Color		
	Round	Pear	Oblong	Orange	Yellow	Green
Oranges	★			★		
Tangerines	★			★		
Bananas			★		★	
Pears		★			★	
Kiwi	★					★

If you were more comfortable learning the information about fruit from the two paragraphs of text, place an **X** next to the "L" below. If the table appealed to you more, place an **X** next to the "R". If you are equally comfortable with both, place an **X** next to the "I" (integrated).

_____ "L"   _____ "I"   _____ "R"

2.   Picture the following scenario: You are going downtown to do some errands. Your errands will require you to go to the bank, the post office, the hardware store, the gas station, and the grocery store. The location of each facility is as follows:

◆ Bank

                                          ◆ Gas Station

                        ◆ Grocery Store

◆ Hardware Store

                                          ◆ Post Office

                  ◆◆ Your Home

If, either before leaving the house or while you were driving, you would think about the sequence in which you plan to do the errands in the most efficient way, place an **X** next to the "L". If you would complete the errands in a random order, place an **X** next to the "R". If sometimes you would plan and sometimes you would not, place an **X** next to the "I".

_____ "L"   _____ "I"   _____ "R"

Learning Environment

The following checklist, although by no means complete, can help you identify the learning environment best suited for your concentration and learning needs. Place a check mark in the boxes next to the items that you prefer.

Individual Preferences		
☐ Morning	☐ Afternoon	☐ Evening
☐ Quiet	☐ Soft Music	☐ Noisy
☐ Sitting	☐ Standing	☐ Moving
☐ Snacking	☐ Talking	☐ Writing
☐ Typing	☐ Colorful Room	☐ Muted Tones
☐ Alone	☐ Partner	☐ Group

Partner/Group Preferences		
Frequency of Meetings	☐ Regularly ☐ Often	☐ As Needed
Duration of Sessions	☐ One Hour ☐ Two Hours	☐ Flexible
Structure	☐ Hierarchical ☐ Participative	☐ Debate

Learning Profile Application

After progressing through the three learning style exercises, you may be wondering how this information can be utilized to assist you with your preparation for the Physical Therapist Examination. Each of the learning style activities provides unique insight into your individual learning style.

The knowledge acquired about your input and processing needs can be utilized as a guide to design your study schedule to suit your Active/Passive preferences. For example, if you have identified that you prefer to be active at input, you intentionally can incorporate visual, auditory, and/or tactile-kinesthetic stimulation into your study sessions. Let's assume that you are reviewing orthopedic special tests. The visual channel can be activated by reading orthopedic textbooks, examining pictures, or watching videotapes of selected special tests. The auditory channel can be activated by listening to yourself or others talk about selected special tests, and the tactile/kinesthetic channel can be utilized by performing selected special tests on another individual.

This same approach can be utilized regardless of the material being reviewed or relearned. It is probably not realistic for individuals always to plan learning experiences based solely on their learning style preferences; however, consistent use of a preferred learning style will tend to maximize a candidate's efficiency during his/her preparation for the Physical Therapist Examination.

The knowledge acquired about your learning environment preferences can assist you in creating a productive study atmosphere when working alone or with others. It also can assist you in selecting an appropriate study partner and/or indicate whether you are a good candidate for group learning.

The knowledge acquired about thinking mode preferences will apply directly to the questions on the Physical Therapist Examination. Since the examination emphasizes clinically oriented material, it requires integrated thinking. Candidates must not only know cognitive information, but they must also demonstrate performance proficiency. Suggestions for an effective information gathering system to achieve integration will be presented in Unit Five.

If you determined you were left-brain dominant on the thinking mode exercise, you probably will be more comfortable answering questions that demonstrate more of a left-brain bias. Conversely, if you are right-brain dominant, you probably will be more comfortable answering questions that demonstrate more of a right-brain bias. Examination questions, although usually requiring integrated thinking, still may have a left or right-brain bias. By being familiar with the characteristics of both left and right-brain questions, candidates can develop an increased awareness of their own learning style and develop particular learning activities directed toward their non-dominant thinking mode.

Exercise

The following exercise provides three sample questions. As you read each of the questions, take note of those which are easy for you and those which are more of a challenge, and see if you can determine why. A brief analysis of each question is presented, along with an answer key at the conclusion of the exercise.

Each of the answer keys throughout the text lists the best answer to each question and identifies a resource which supports the stated answer. In the vast majority of cases a page number is also provided to direct candidates to the appropriate subject matter. The complete reference for each of the resources is located in the bibliography.

Sample Question One

Based on the "rule of nines", an adult who has burns over her anterior right arm, the anterior portion of the thorax, and the genital region would be classified as having burns over _____ percent of her body?

1. 19
2. 22.5
3. 23.5
4. 28

Analysis

This question will tend to favor left-brain dominant candidates. The question requires candidates to recall detailed information, specifically the percentage of total body surface allocated to the nine various anatomical segments.

Sample Question Two

A therapist observes a client ambulating in the physical therapy gym. The therapist notes that the client's pelvis drops on the right during left stance phase. In an attempt to compensate, the client laterally bends his trunk over the stance leg. This type of gait deviation can be caused by weakness of the _____?

1. gluteus maximus
2. gluteus medius
3. iliopsoas
4. tensor fasciae latae

Analysis

This question will tend to favor right-brain dominant candidates. The question requires candidates to identify the relationship between specific muscle function and a resultant gait deviation.

Sample Question Three

A physical therapist is treating a six month old infant with spina bifida. The infant suddenly begins to act strangely during the treatment session. A primary survey reveals the infant is not breathing, but does have a pulse. The most immediate response would be to _____?

1. begin chest compressions
2. begin mouth to mouth breathing
3. begin mouth to nose breathing
4. begin mouth to mouth and nose breathing

Analysis

This question is more representative of the integrated type that will make up the majority of the Physical Therapist Examination. This specific question requires candidates not only to be familiar with the sequential steps of cardiopulmonary resuscitation, but also to recognize the relationship among a number of other factors including when a client has a pulse and is not breathing. The candidate further is required to identify the most immediate response.

Answer Key

1. Answer: 3   Resource: O'Sullivan (515)

   The percentage of body surface burned in an adult can be calculated using the rule of nines: anterior right arm 4.5%, anterior portion of the thorax 18%, genital region 1%. Total = 23.5%

2. Answer: 2   Resource: Magee (690)

   The gluteus medius muscle is a hip abductor. Weakness of the abductor can result in a Trendelenburg gait.

3. Answer: 4   Resource: National Safety Council (32)
                                                First Aid & CPR

   Mouth to mouth and nose breathing is utilized on an infant (under 1 year).

As you progress through the sample questions in this text, it should become apparent that to be successful on the examination, a candidate will have to demonstrate both left and right-brain proficiency. It is therefore advisable for a candidate's study plan to incorporate activities which utilize both left-brain and right-brain thinking modes.

We will continue to expand on many of the topics we have introduced throughout the text. Included in the following unit will be general and specific study guidelines and specific learning style recommendations.

Unit Four
Study Plan

The simple thought of preparing for a comprehensive examination such as the Physical Therapist Examination can be overwhelming. Many candidates ask themselves how it is possible to prepare adequately for an examination that encompasses more than two years of professional coursework.

One of the largest advantages of taking an examination such as the Physical Therapist Examination is that it does not require candidates to demonstrate mastery of new material. On the surface this may not seem like a significant advantage, but since candidates are, in effect, only reviewing or relearning previously presented information, their level of attainment should be significantly greater.

Many candidates fail to utilize this advantage. Candidates who attempt to learn large quantities of new information, instead of focusing on understanding and applying basic concepts, often do themselves a tremendous disservice. It is true that there undoubtedly will be questions that contain information that was not part of a selected curriculum, but to attempt to study this new information would be a large mistake for most candidates. Instead, candidates should focus on reviewing or relearning basic concepts that are an integral component of all accredited physical therapy programs. It is this type of information that will make up the vast majority of the examination. Individuals who take this common sense approach optimize their chances of success on this important examination.

Developing a Plan

Developing a study plan allows candidates to take control of their preparation. Candidates should begin by compiling a list of all the necessary topics that must be reviewed prior to the examination. The topics should be assembled in a sequence that will allow for a smooth transition between topics. Candidates should make an estimate of the time needed to review each topic and compile a list of available resources.

The Reporter's Formula

Throughout history, individuals have been sent out to gather information about ideas, events, processes and people. To assist these individuals, a specific formula was developed. This formula was termed "the reporter's formula."

The reporter's formula contains the following seven question words: Who, What, Which, When, Where, How, and Why. This time tested technique of information gathering can be utilized by candidates preparing for the Physical Therapist Examination in a number of different ways:

1. Incorporate the formula into a study plan for each content category
2. Utilize the formula as an outline for study sessions
3. Generate potential examination questions using the formula

The formula also can be used to categorize actual examination questions. This specific technique will be explored in detail in Unit Five.

Question Words

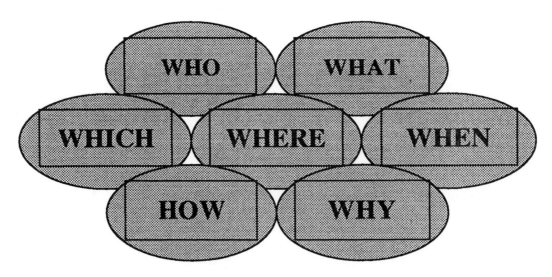

Goals

Before beginning to study, develop specific goals for each study session. Ideally, these goals should be established on a weekly basis. Establishing goals will ensure that candidates cover the desired material and will serve as a mechanism to keep them on schedule with their study plan. Candidates should be realistic with the goals they establish and should not attempt to cover more material than is possible in a particular study session.

Reviewing

Reviewing is defined operationally as looking over or studying previously learned information. Reviewing can play an important role in a candidate's preparation for the Physical Therapist Examination. It is recommended that students review classnotes for their practice oriented professional coursework. Practice oriented professional coursework typically includes, but is not limited to, study of the musculoskeletal, cardiopulmonary, and neurosensory systems. In addition, candidates usually have coursework in client care skills, physical agents, administration, ethics, research and education. Each of these topics are important components of the content outline for the Physical Therapist Examination.

Classnotes may seem voluminous to candidates, but they can be reviewed fairly quickly. Special attention must be taken not to become bogged down in one specific area for any significant amount of time. General concepts that are understood should be scanned quickly, while other concepts that are more difficult for a candidate should be read carefully. Concepts that remain unclear after being reviewed should be written down for future study sessions.

Other foundational coursework encountered earlier in the professional curriculum can be consulted as needed during various study sessions. This type of coursework often includes, but is not limited to Anatomy and Physiology, Neuroanatomy, Exercise Physiology, and Kinesiology. It is important to limit the amount of time spent reviewing this type of foundational coursework. Candidates often can make better use of their allotted time by reviewing coursework encountered later in the curriculum that may be more practice oriented. By reviewing practice oriented information, candidates not only keep their studying consistent with the format of the examination, but at the same time indirectly review much of the information presented in the foundational coursework.

Relearning

Relearning is defined operationally as reacquiring knowledge or comprehension which was known previously. Relearning is often a necessary component of a comprehensive study plan. In physical therapy academic programs, candidates constantly are learning new information on a variety of topics. Although students typically exhibit mastery of selected material during a scheduled examination, they do not always retain the information for later use. The failure to retain information that was learned previously is the primary rationale for relearning.

Relearning can take place in a variety of ways. Often times, simply reviewing information is enough for candidates to relearn the material; however, in some cases, a more in-depth approach is necessary. This approach may include using textbooks, class handouts and interacting with classmates or professors. It is imperative that candidates relearn material which may be an integral component of the examination. It must be stressed, however, that to focus on memorizing minuscule facts or inordinate details would be, at best, poor utilization of available study time.

Journal

It is recommended that candidates keep a daily journal of their studying. This journal should include a variety of information:

1. Topics/concepts that were reviewed successfully
2. Topics/concepts requiring additional review or relearning
3. List of goals for each study session
4. Progress towards meeting established goals
5. Resources utilized during the study session
6. Plan for the subsequent study session

As candidates begin to complete sample examinations, the journal will allow them to document specific information on their performance. This should include the percentage of questions answered correctly and the amount of time necessary to complete a selected examination. Candidates should survey questions that were answered incorrectly and attempt to determine if there are any general patterns. For example, if a candidate consistently has difficulty answering questions related to a specific topic area or questions that were constructed in a similar manner, these deficits should be recorded. Once identified, appropriate remedial strategies can be developed.

General Recommendations

To this point, candidates have learned a variety of strategies to utilize when developing a study plan for the Physical Therapist Examination. There are, however, a variety of other variables which can influence the quality of a study session. This text will describe many of these variables.

Environment

To construct an optimal learning environment, candidates should attempt to incorporate their individual learning preferences into each study session. Return to Unit Three to re-examine the preferences best suited for your specific concentration and learning needs.

Supplies

Gather the necessary supplies to assist you in studying. Begin the study session with all of the supplies necessary to complete the entire session. Unnecessary breaks to gather additional resources will serve only to prolong or limit the effectiveness of your study session.

Timing

We all function more effectively at specific times of the day. Ideally, study sessions should take place when the mind is alert and attentive. Select a time during the day when you feel you are at your optimal level of functioning. Avoid studying when you are physically tired. Activities such as eating or heavy exercise can lead to decreased attentiveness, and as a result, decrease the effectiveness of your study session.

Make sure your emotional state is conducive to learning. If you have had a particularly bad day, avoid studying. Study sessions tend to be unproductive when a candidate is less than 100 percent emotionally.

Frequency and Duration

Studying for short intervals of time has proven to be a more effective learning strategy than studying for long intervals. Specific parameters for frequency and duration are not provided, since they can vary considerably for different learning styles and purposes.

Partnership and Group Recommendations

Many candidates can significantly enhance their preparation for the Physical Therapist Examination by participating in a study partnership or group. This type of collaboration can offer candidates several distinct benefits:

1. Candidates can learn from the information presented by others and as a result, can often reduce their individual study time.

2. Candidates can receive assistance from others when remediation is necessary.

3. Candidates can assess and modify their individual study plan based on the perceptions and knowledge of others.

Although these arrangements have the potential to be a valuable component of a comprehensive study plan, they need to be structured in a fashion that will allow candidates to be productive. Failure to have adequate structure often can result in a study session degenerating into a purely social event. To avoid this potential pitfall, we recommend the following guidelines for all partnerships or groups:

1. Set rules of behavior and a method for staying on task.

2. Set the length and frequency of study sessions, keeping in mind your long range plan.

3. Set goals that indicate the amount of material to be covered in a specified time period.

4. Establish time during scheduled study sessions to address individual learning needs.

5. Discuss and agree on an agenda for each scheduled study session.

6. Decide on the structure of each study session:

hierarchical	someone acts as "teacher" for each session
participative	each member acts as facilitator for an area of study
debate	exchange of ideas after independent study

7. Attempt to institute a firm schedule for study sessions and emphasize the importance of attendance at each session.

8. Decide on the learning tools the partnership/group will use during each study session.

Learning Style

The following section offers candidates specific recommendations based on their individual input/processing preferences. Candidates should attempt to utilize this information when participating in a study partnership or group.

Active/Active

Format

Study sessions should consist of 60-90 minutes of interactive study. The sessions should be designed based on the categories contained within the content outline. Candidates should divide the content outline into smaller, more manageable components.

Many active learners will find it helpful to develop three specific concepts, ideas, or processes to work on for each scheduled study session. After the study session is completed, candidates should make sure they have achieved each established goal. Ample time should be allotted at the end of the study session for a brief review.

Active/Active learners often prefer to divide the workload for the next session. These tasks typically are done independently and usually involve reviewing selected material that will be discussed as part of the next session. This same routine can be repeated with each study session until the actual examination.

Group Composition

Group members should include learners who are active for input, or processing, or both. There should be a representative sample of left-brain (facts, details) and right-brain (big picture, relationships) dominant candidates.

Frequency

Since multisensory stimulation is more difficult to achieve alone, it is recommended that study sessions take place as frequently as possible. Daily study sessions would not be considered excessive.

Concerns

Effective time management is critical, because it can take considerably longer to achieve multisensory stimulation.

Learning Tools

Color-coding may help in stimulating the visual channel. Discussions, simulations, hands-on practice and role playing are viable learning activities.

        Left-brain: lists, outlines, flow charts
        Right-brain: charts, graphs, mind maps

Tips

Position yourself so that you can observe body language during the study session. Videotapes of sessions may be useful to play back during individual study time to help recreate the study session.

Active/Passive

Format

Study sessions should be scheduled for a maximum of two hours. The sessions should be designed based on the categories contained within the content outline. Candidates should divide the content outline into smaller, more manageable components.

Many active learners will find it helpful to develop three specific concepts, ideas or processes to work on for each scheduled study session. After the study session is completed, candidates should make sure they have achieved each established goal.

Ample time should be allotted at the end of the study session for a brief review, and specific tasks should be delegated for the following study session. These tasks typically are done independently and usually involve reviewing selected material that will be discussed as part of the next study session. This same routine can be repeated with each study session until the actual examination.

Although most Active/Passive learners prefer to review information themselves, we recommend that they use a participative format for group work. In this format, each member assumes responsibility for an area of study. Group activity will limit the detailed studying these learners prefer, and provide them with a more comprehensive understanding of the presented material.

Group Composition

Group members should include learners who are active for input, or processing, or both. There should be a representative sample of left-brain (facts, details) and right-brain (big picture, relationships) dominant candidates.

Frequency

Two to three times per week is recommended. Candidates may have a desire to reduce the number of sessions; however, they are best served by frequent meetings.

Concerns

Time management is necessary to maintain concentration and allow for a smooth progression through the content outline.

Learning Tools

Color-coding may help in stimulating the visual channel. Discussions, simulations, hands-on practice, role playing, and blackboard "teaching" are viable examples.

Left-brain:	lists, outlines, flow charts
Right-brain:	charts, graphs, mind maps

Tips

Position yourself so that you can observe body language during the study session. Videotapes of sessions may be useful to play back during individual study time to help recreate the study session.

Passive/Active

Format

Since the majority of studying will take place independently, study sessions should function as an opportunity for candidates to assess their current study plan and benefit from the knowledge of others.

Study sessions should range from two to three hours in length and should focus on large pieces of material. An example of this would be a session at the conclusion of a major section of the content outline.

Group Composition

Group members should include learners who prefer to study alone and then gather to discuss specific information. Both left and right-brain dominant candidates should be included in the group.

Frequency

Approximately once per week is recommended. This schedule will allow candidates to cover the necessary material within the established time parameters.

Concerns

Since the majority of studying has been completed before the review sessions, candidates need to be very careful to include both concepts and applications in their study plan.

Learning Tools

Blackboard presentations, briefings, debate, occasional simulations.

> Left-brain: outlines, lists, flow charts
> Right-brain: charts, graphs, mind maps

Tips

Candidates may have little patience with partners or group members who come to sessions unprepared.

Passive/Passive

Format

Since the majority of studying will take place independently, study sessions should function as an opportunity for candidates to assess their current study plan and benefit from the knowledge of others.

Study sessions should range from two to three hours in length and should focus on large pieces of material. An example of this would be a session at the conclusion of a major section of the content outline. Since candidates' focus in this category is not on application of material, they should make sure that this area is addressed at each study session.

Group Composition

Group members should include individuals who prefer to study alone initially. The group should also include members who are application driven.

Frequency

Approximately once per week is recommended. This schedule will allow candidates to cover the necessary material within the established time parameters.

Concerns

Time management is necessary to maintain concentration and limit the role of stress.

Learning Tools

Lectures, blackboard presentations, briefings, observation of simulations, handouts, texts, notes.

> Left-brain: outlines, lists, flow charts
> Right-brain: charts, graphs, mind maps

Tips

Passive/Passive learners may become very uncomfortable physically engaging in learning activities before having a chance to review and observe.

Unit Five
Multiple Choice Examinations

Do you believe that Mark McGwire was hitting 500 foot homeruns as a little leaguer or that Martina Hingis was consistently hitting blistering passing shots in the second grade? Your answer to these questions is likely to be no. Since history tells us these individuals later accomplished the aforementioned feats, the question becomes, what allowed these individuals to progress to such lofty heights?

The answer probably can best be described in a single word, "practice." Surely individuals like Mark McGwire and Martina Hingis were blessed with certain athletic and physical traits which allowed them the opportunity to become successful, but it was their dedication, desire, and determination that allowed them to evolve into superstars in their respective fields.

In physical therapy, there are an abundance of skills that must be learned by the entry level practitioner. Mastery of these skills often requires physical therapists to demonstrate the same type of dedication, desire, and determination exhibited by Mark McGwire and Martina Hingis.

Test taking skills are specific skills which allow individuals to utilize the characteristics and format of a selected examination in order to maximize their performance. These skills can be very valuable when taking an examination such as the Physical Therapist Examination. Despite the importance of this topic, very little, if any, academic time is set aside to address test taking skills. The good news is that test taking skills can be learned and that through dedication, desire, and determination, these skills can serve effectively to improve your performance on this important examination.

Since the Physical Therapist Examination utilizes a multiple choice format, further discussion of test taking skills will be solely concerned with this particular format. Test taking skills can allow candidates to increase their ability to recognize cues within the multiple choice question. These cues can be utilized to provide valuable information towards identifying the correct response. It has been documented in the literature that recognition of selected cues can lead to improved examination scores.

Individuals who are able to recognize such cues are said to be "test wise." Perhaps this explains, in part, why many students who have prepared adequately for a selected examination often perform poorly. Test taking skills are acquired skills that develop with practice. This unit will present candidates with valuable information on multiple choice examinations and a variety of test taking skills. The unit also will provide candidates with an opportunity to apply the described test taking skills on selected sample examination questions.

Multiple Choice Questions

The Physical Therapist Examination is a 200 question multiple choice examination. The objective examination consists of multiple choice questions with four potentially correct answers to each question. Candidates are instructed to select the "best answer" to complete each question.

Before we begin to explore selected test taking strategies, we need to identify the various components of a multiple choice question. Multiple choice questions can be dissected into specific identifiable components:

Item	An item refers to an individual multiple choice question and the corresponding potential answers.
Stem	The stem refers to the statement that asks the question.
Options	Options refer to the potential answers to the question asked. One option in each item will be the "best answer," while the others are distracters.

Item

The Physical Therapist Examination contains 200 items. Each item consists of a stem and four options. Items may vary considerably in content and length, but should utilize a consistent format.

Stem

The stem can take on a variety of forms. Typically, the stem conveys to the reader the necessary information needed to respond correctly to the question. In addition to the necessary information, many times extraneous information also is included in the stem. This information, when not recognized by the candidate as unnecessary, often can act as a significant distracter.

The stem commonly can take on the form of a complete sentence, an incomplete sentence, or a fill-in-the-blank. The stem can be expressed in a positive or negative form. A positive form would require a candidate to identify correct information, while a negative form would require a candidate to identify incorrect information. It is important to scrutinize each stem, since a single key word such as "not" or "except" can turn a positive stem into a negative stem. Failure to identify this can lead to the identification of an incorrect answer.

Options

Options can take on a variety of forms, including a single word, a group of words, an incomplete sentence, a complete sentence, or a group of sentences. The method for analyzing each option does not change, regardless of form.

Question Categorization System

Let's take a few moments to review what we already have learned about the Physical Therapist Examination. We know that the examination consists of 200 multiple choice questions, each with four possible options. We also know that each question will be representative of one of the three content areas identified in the content outline.

As we introduced in Unit Four, the reporter's formula can be a valuable tool to assist candidates with their preparation for the examination. The reporter's formula utilizes seven specific question words: Who, What, Which, Where, When, How and Why. By relating each of the question words to the material in the content outline, candidates can effectively review the majority of the information that will be encountered on the Physical Therapist Examination. By reviewing the information in this manner, therapists gather and store the information in an organized and efficient fashion.

This system also can be utilized to a candidate's advantage when analyzing a multiple choice question. As candidates analyze specific examination questions, they should attempt to categorize each question using the same seven question words. By identifying the correct question word for each of the multiple choice questions, candidates are, in effect, telling the brain where to access the desired information. Since a candidate's study plan was designed in a similar fashion, this process will improve the rate and fluidity of information retrieval. On a timed examination such as the Physical Therapist Examination, this can be a significant advantage.

It is important for candidates to remember that the purpose of the question categorization system is to assist candidates in understanding the intended meaning of each question. By understanding exactly what each question is asking, candidates can avoid making careless mistakes and improve their examination performance.

Four Levels of Learning
&
Related Question Types

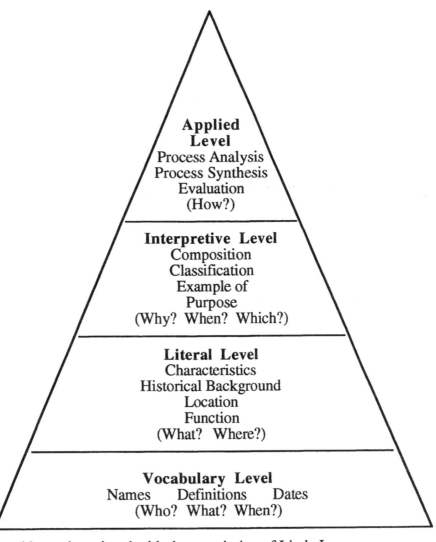

Applied Level
Process Analysis
Process Synthesis
Evaluation
(How?)

Interpretive Level
Composition
Classification
Example of
Purpose
(Why? When? Which?)

Literal Level
Characteristics
Historical Background
Location
Function
(What? Where?)

Vocabulary Level
Names   Definitions   Dates
(Who? What? When?)

Figure adapted by and reprinted with the permission of Linda Lyon.

Of course, we have oversimplified the process, but in your mind you should begin to see how this information can be applied effectively to the Physical Therapist Examination.

In an attempt to allow candidates to accurately classify examination items, we have divided the seven question words into five separate categories. Selected sample examination questions will be offered to illustrate the use of each category.

Each item in this section will deal with vital signs. Remember, to be classified into a specific category, the exact question word associated with the category does not have to be utilized; rather, think in terms of the problem solving process or the information required to answer the question.

Exercise

Answer each sample question using the provided answer space. An answer key is located at the conclusion of the exercise.

Who

This category contains information concerning specific individuals who have made various contributions to the field of physical therapy. It also could include information related to a specific discipline or the responsibilities associated with the discipline.

Sample Question

1. A physical therapist works on an interdisciplinary team in an acute care hospital. One of the clients scheduled to be treated has had severe fluctuations in her blood pressure throughout the night and has been monitored by the nursing staff. Which interdisciplinary team member would be the most appropriate to determine the client's ability to complete her scheduled rehabilitative session?

    1. physical therapist
    2. occupational therapist
    3. nurse
    4. physician

What/Which

This category contains information associated with facts and details. To learn this information typically requires memorization.

What/Which information can be divided into five separate categories:

- Definition
- Characteristics
- Classification
- Composition
- Example

Definition
> meanings of words, terms or procedures

Sample Question

2. A therapist reviews the medical record of a client scheduled to be examined in physical therapy. An entry in the medical record indicates the client has tachycardia. Which description most accurately defines tachycardia?

   1. an abnormally fast heart rate
   2. an abnormally slow heart rate
   3. shortness of breath
   4. labored or difficult breathing

Characteristics
> distinguishing traits, qualities, or properties

Sample Question

3. A therapist records the vital signs of a 42 year old female at rest. The client was referred to physical therapy after sustaining a trimalleolar fracture. Which of the following values would not be considered within normal limits?

   1. pulse: 82 beats per minute
   2. blood pressure: 128/85 mm Hg
   3. respiration rate: 20 respirations per minute
   4. body temperature: 97.8 °F

Classification
> arranging in, or assigning to, various groups, classes or categories

Sample Question

4. A therapist measures the blood pressure of a 68 year old male. The therapist determines the client's blood pressure is 128/84 mm Hg. This can best be classified as _____?

   1. mild hypotension
   2. mild hypertension
   3. moderate hypertension
   4. within normal limits

Composition
> identifying individual elements or arrangements

Sample Question

5. A therapist attempts to calculate a client's age predicted maximum heart rate. Which of the following is utilized as a component of the age predicted maximum heart rate formula?

   1. 180
   2. 200
   3. 220
   4. 240

Example
   a representative sample

Sample Question

6. There are many factors that can influence blood pressure. Which of the following would tend to increase resting blood pressure?

   1. medication
   2. anxiety
   3. loss of blood
   4. decreased cardiac output

Where

Information in this category usually refers to a location.

Sample Question

7. A therapist assesses a client's pulse. In order to accurately assess the client's apical pulse, the therapist should position the stethoscope _____?

   1. on the chest wall over the apex of the heart
   2. over the femoral artery
   3. over the carotid artery
   4. over the posterior tibial artery

As you can see by answering the Who, What, Which, and Where questions for each of the content areas, there will be very little information that will be omitted from your review. However, you also should recognize that the majority of the material contained within these question words has dealt with fact based information and has not emphasized clinical application. The next series of categories will be more prevalent on the Physical Therapist Examination. They will deal almost exclusively with clinical application.

How/When

Information in this category involves processes; specifically how to perform tasks step by step and how to analyze what has been done. In some cases, the information follows a sequential timeline (whole-to-part) and sometimes it necessitates drawing together diverse information (part-to-whole) and forming a conclusion.

How/When information can be divided into two categories:

- Process Analysis
- Process Synthesis

Process Analysis
step by step sequencing of information or actions

Sample Question

8. A client sitting in a chair in the physical therapy waiting room suddenly falls to the floor and appears to be unconscious. The therapist determines that the client is not breathing and administers two rescue breaths. The therapist then checks the client's carotid pulse. If the therapist is able to detect a pulse, he/she should next _____?

   1. begin external chest compressions
   2. continue rescue breathing
   3. readjust the head tilt and attempt to ventilate
   4. determine the pulse rate for 60 seconds

Process Synthesis
merging of information into "the big picture" and making an informed "action plan"

Sample Question

9. A client with quadriplegia is two weeks status post cervical spinal fusion. After transferring the client from bed to a wheelchair, the client complains of a severe headache. Upon examination, the client is found to be diaphoretic and flushed. The client's blood pressure is recorded as 210/130 mmHg. These signs and symptoms are most indicative of _____?

   1. autonomic dysreflexia
   2. urinary tract infection
   3. orthostatic hypotension
   4. pulmonary embolus

Why

This category typically requires a more advanced level of knowledge than many of the other categories. To answer a Why question successfully, it may be necessary to answer simultaneously What, Which, Where and/or How information.

Why information can be divided into two categories:

- Cause and Effect
- Function/Use Concepts

Cause and Effect
relationship between an outcome or state of being and the causative factors

Sample Question

10. A therapist attempts to assess the blood pressure of a grossly obese client. If the bladder of the blood pressure cuff used is too narrow in relation to the circumference of the client's arm, which of the following would best describe the resultant effect on the client's measured blood pressure?

    1. the value will be erroneously low
    2. the value will be erroneously high
    3. the value will be reflective of the client's actual blood pressure
    4. the value will not be reflective of the client's actual blood pressure

Function/Use Concepts
explanation or rationale for a selected action

Sample Question

11. A therapist establishes a baseline measurement of a client's vital signs prior to beginning a phase II cardiac rehabilitation program. The primary purpose of conducting the baseline measurement is to _____?

    1. determine the therapeutic measures most appropriate to the client's rehabilitation program
    2. demonstrate objective progress in the client's rehabilitation program
    3. protect the therapist from unnecessary litigation
    4. identify significant changes in the values as a result of exercise or other factors

It is possible that many of the examination questions will fall into more than one of the question categories. Therefore, it is important for candidates to be judicious in the amount of time allotted to determining the best category for each question.

Answer Key

1. Answer: 4   Resource: Guide for Professional Conduct

   Severe fluctuations in blood pressure can be indicative of a serious medical condition. The physician is the appropriate professional to assess the client's changing medical status.

2. Answer: 1   Resource: Minor (39)

   Tachycardia is an abnormally fast heart rate, greater than 100 beats per minute.

3. Answer: 3   Resource: Pierson (59)

   Normal respiration rate in an adult is 12-18 breaths per minute.

4. Answer: 4   Resource: Minor (42)

   128/84 mmHg is within the accepted blood pressure range for adults.

5. Answer: 3   Resource: Kisner (137)

   Age predicted maximum heart rate is defined as (220-age).

6. Answer: 2   Resource: Pierson (59)

   Blood pressure will increase with anxiety and other significant changes in emotional status.

7. Answer: 1   Resource: Pierson (47)

   Auscultation over the apex of the heart using a stethoscope can be used to assess the apical pulse.

8. Answer: 2   Resource: National Safety Council (26)

   Rescue breathing is indicated for a client that is not breathing, however does have a detectable pulse.

9. Answer: 1   Resource: Pierson (335)

   Autonomic dysreflexia is an exaggerated reflex of the autonomic nervous system. It often occurs in individuals with recent spinal cord injuries and is characterized by severe hypertension, headache, and sweating.

10. Answer: 2   Resource: Pierson (56)

    A narrow blood pressure cuff will cause the measured value to be high. The width of the bladder should be 40% of the circumference of the midpoint of the limb.

11. Answer: 4   Resource: Brannon (250)

Significant changes in vital signs can only be determined when compared to baseline values. This is a fundamental component of all cardiac rehabilitation programs.

Task Approach

On the Physical Therapist Examination there are 200 items that candidates must answer within a four hour time period. Due to the length of the examination and the time constraints associated with it, candidates need to approach the examination in a systematic and organized fashion. Loss of control during the examination typically will yield poor results that are not reflective of a candidate's actual knowledge. We will introduce a four phase process as an example of an approach that can be used effectively when answering examination questions in a review text or on a computer.

Phase I

Carefully read the stem of the first item. Underline key words or groups of words that offer valuable information. Circle command words that indicate the desired action. If, after reading the stem, you are able to generate an answer to the item, make a mental note or write the hypothesized answer on scratch paper.

Candidates should then begin to examine each option one at a time. It is important to read the entire option, since one word often can make a potentially correct answer incorrect. If the generated answer is consistent with one of the available options, the candidate should give the option strong consideration; however since more than one option can be correct it is imperative to analyze each presented option. If candidates are not able to generate a response, regardless of the reason, they should place an asterisk next to the item number and move to the next item.

Since computer based testing does not allow candidates to mark desired words or phrases, they need to make use of several less direct indicators. These indicators usually take the form of a mental note or a brief written message.

Phase II

Once candidates have completed all of the questions to which they can generate an answer, they should progress to a true/false format. This format allows candidates to have only one potential option in front of them at a time; therefore significantly limiting the distracters.

Candidates should begin by uncovering one of the available options and saying to themselves, "Is it true that ...?" Be sure to substitute the key terms and command words from the stem. Place a "T" or "F" next to the selected option and move to the next option. Continue this pattern until all of the available options have been analyzed. If, after applying this technique, an answer becomes apparent, the candidate should select the answer. If the answer is not apparent, the candidate should move to the next question.

Phase III

By the time a candidate progresses to this phase, the vast majority of the questions on the examination should have been answered. Candidates should return to the beginning of the examination and revisit each remaining question with an asterisk. Candidates again should attempt to generate a response to each of the questions. Likewise, candidates should attempt to analyze unanswered questions by revisiting the true/false format.

Phase IV

At this point there should be very few remaining unanswered questions. Candidates now must utilize deductive reasoning strategies to answer the remaining questions. Deductive reasoning strategies allow candidates to secure points beyond those acquired through direct knowledge of subject matter. Although deductive reasoning strategies are not meant to be used in place of academic knowledge, they have proven to be an effective strategy to improve examination performance.

Deductive reasoning strategies often allow candidates to eliminate one or more of the potential answers. Elimination of any option significantly increases the probability of identifying the correct answer. On the Physical Therapist Examination, eliminating one option increases the chance of selecting a correct answer from 25% to 33%. Eliminating two options increases the chance of selecting a correct answer to 50%. Although on the surface this may not seem terribly significant, on a test such as the Physical Therapist Examination, where there are 200 questions, this can be the difference between a passing and a failing score. Selected deductive reasoning strategies that can be used effectively on the Physical Therapist Examination are presented.

Absurd Options

Many times a multiple choice item will include an option that is not consistent with what the stem is asking or with the other options. In many cases, this option can be eliminated. Rapid elimination of specific options will allow candidates to spend additional time analyzing other possible options.

Similar Options

When two or more options have a similar meaning or express the same fact, they often imply each other's incorrectness. Since candidates taking the Physical Therapist Examination are instructed to select the best answer, it would be extremely unlikely that one of two options that are so close in resemblance would be the correct answer. For this reason, candidates can often eliminate both options.

Obtainable Information

There is a great deal of factual material that candidates must sift through when taking the Physical Therapist Examination. In some instances, the material can provide candidates with valuable information that can assist them in answering other examination questions.

Errors in Test Construction

Since many different individuals are involved in developing the Physical Therapist

Examination, it is difficult to make generalizations about examination construction. Candidates should attempt to answer each question exactly as it is written and avoid the temptation to speculate on the intention of the item's author.

Degree of Qualification

Particularly in the sciences, there seem to be many exceptions to general rules. Therefore, specific determiners such as "always" or "never" often overqualify an option. Research indicates that more general options are the correct answer a significantly higher percentage of the time.

Position of the Correct Answer

Research has demonstrated the tendency for the correct answer in a sequence of alternatives to be at the center of the response distribution. On the Physical Therapist Examination, the center of the response distribution would correlate to answers 2 and 3.

It is important to remember that deductive reasoning strategies should not be used as a substitute for academic knowledge. Deductive reasoning strategies, when applied indiscriminately or as a substitute for academic knowledge, lead to poor results. Deductive reasoning strategies should be applied only when candidates are unable to identify the correct response using academic knowledge. In these instances, deductive reasoning strategies can be used in combination with academic knowledge to increase the probability of selecting the best answer to a specific examination item.

If, after progressing through the four phase process, a candidate still is unable to make an informed decision, he/she should simply attempt to guess at the correct answer. Since there is no penalty associated with guessing on the Physical Therapist Examination, it is in a candidate's best interest to answer each question.

Exercise

In this exercise, three sample questions are presented. Candidates should attempt to identify the best answer to each question by utilizing the four phase process. Candidates should also attempt to identify the question type and the specific content area.

The following tables list the possible responses in each category:

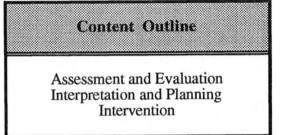

Question Category	Content Outline
Who What/Which Where How/When Why	Assessment and Evaluation Interpretation and Planning Intervention

An analysis section immediately follows each of the three sample questions. The analysis section begins by showing the sample question with key terms underlined and command words in bold type. A brief narrative follows, which describes how the four phase process can be applied to the sample question.

An answer key, located at the conclusion of the exercise, indicates the best answer, question type, and content category for each of the sample questions.

Sample Question One

A therapist instructs a client with a Foley catheter in ambulation activities. During ambulation the therapist should position the collection bag _____?

1. above the level of the client's bladder
2. below the level of the client's bladder
3. above the level of the client's heart
4. below the level of the client's heart

Analysis

A therapist instructs a client with a <u>Foley catheter in ambulation activities</u>. During ambulation the therapist should **position** <u>the collection bag _____</u>?

1. above the level of the client's bladder
2. below the level of the client's bladder
3. above the level of the client's heart
4. below the level of the client's heart

After reading the stem and identifying the pertinent information a candidate should attempt to generate an answer. The candidate then should begin to reveal each of the available options. If a generated answer is consistent with one of the available options, there is a high probability that the answer is correct.

If a candidate was not able to generate an answer, he/she should progress to a true/false format. The candidate will begin this process by creating a true/false statement for each of the available options. The true/false statement for option "1" would be as follows:

Is it true that during ambulation the therapist should position the collection bag above the level of the client's bladder?

The candidate should answer each question by placing a "T" or "F" next to the corresponding option. He/she should then progress through all of the remaining options in the same manner. Remember, it is possible to have more than one option which satisfactorily answers the question. It is then the candidate's responsibility to select the best answer from the remaining options.

Sample Question Two

A group of physical therapists attempt to determine the relationship between two variables on an examination form. Which of the following correlation coefficients would indicate the strongest relationship?

1. +.86
2. +.45
3. -.34
4. -.89

Analysis

A group of physical therapists attempt to determine <u>the relationship between two variables</u> on an examination form. Which of the following <u>correlation coefficients</u> would indicate the **strongest relationship**?

1. +.86
2. +.45
3. -.34
4. -.89

After reading the stem and identifying the pertinent information, a candidate should recognize that it is virtually impossible to generate an answer prior to viewing the available options. A candidate should, however, begin to think about correlation coefficients and determining the strength of the relationship between variables.

The candidate then should begin to expose each of the available options. Since, in this specific example, all of the options are numerical, it will not be particularly helpful to apply a true/false format. Instead, a candidate simply should examine the possible options and attempt to identify the correct response.

Although the four phase process does not directly supply a candidate with the correct response, by carefully reading the stem, a candidate can avoid an unnecessary mistake. In this item, the stem asks the candidate to identify the correlation coefficient that indicates the strongest relationship between the two variables. If a candidate does not read the question carefully, he/she may make an assumption that the stem is asking for the strongest positive relationship and subsequently answer the question incorrectly.

It is important that a candidate answer each item based only on the given information. By making even small assumptions or by not reading each item carefully, a candidate can make careless mistakes.

Sample Question Three

A therapist completes an isokinetic examination on an 18 year old male rehabilitating from a medial meniscectomy. The therapist notes that the client generates 140 ft/lbs of force using the uninvolved quadriceps at 60 degrees per second. Assuming a normal ratio of hamstrings to quadriceps strength, which of the following would be an acceptable hamstrings value at 60 degrees per second?

1.   64 ft/lbs
2.   84 ft/lbs
3.   114 ft/lbs
4.   116 ft/lbs

Analysis

A therapist completes an isokinetic examination on an 18 year old male rehabilitating from a medial meniscectomy. The therapist notes that the client generates 140 ft/lbs of force using the uninvolved quadriceps at 60 degrees per second. Assuming a normal ratio of hamstrings to quadriceps strength, which of the following would be **an acceptable hamstrings value** at 60 degrees per second?

1.   64 ft/lbs
2.   84 ft/lbs
3.   114 ft/lbs
4.   116 ft/lbs

For the purpose of discussion, let's assume a candidate has no idea of the normal ratio of quadriceps/hamstrings strength at 60 degrees/second. Lack of specific academic knowledge will result in a candidate not being able to identify the correct answer using a Phase I, Phase II or Phase III approach. However, by applying a Phase IV approach and utilizing deductive reasoning strategies, a candidate can significantly increase his/her chances of identifying the best answer without applying direct academic knowledge.

In this item, the stem asks a candidate to identify a value which would be representative of a normal quadriceps/hamstrings ratio at 60 degrees/second. As with many measurements in physical therapy, precise normal values are difficult to ascertain, and therefore often are expressed in ranges. By applying this knowledge to the examination item, a candidate should be able to eliminate options 3 and 4. Since options 3 and 4 are so close in value they imply each other's incorrectness. Although in this example deductive reasoning strategies were not able to identify the correct answer, they were able to eliminate two of the four possible options. By eliminating the two options, a candidate now has a 50% chance of identifying the best answer, even without utilizing any direct academic or clinical knowledge.

Answer Key

1. Answer: 2   Resource: Pierson (267)
   Question Type: Where
   Content Area: Intervention

   The effect of gravity necessitates the collection bag being below the level of the client's bladder.

2. Answer: 4   Resource: Currier (265)
   Question Type: Why
   Content Area: Intervention

   Correlation coefficients range from +1.00 to -1.00. Since the question does not ask for a positive or negative correlation, the strongest relationship is indicated by -.89.

3. Answer: 2   Resource: Hamill (236)
   Question Type: Why
   Content Area: Interpretation and Planning

   A gross estimate of quadriceps:hamstrings ratio is 3:2.

We have attempted to illustrate how the four phase process can be applied to a number of different sample questions. Although candidates may not always be able to identify the correct answer using this strategy, when used appropriately, it can serve as a valuable tool to maximize a candidate's performance on the Physical Therapist Examination.

Exercise

The following exercise contains ten sample questions for candidates to answer. Resist the urge to approach the questions in a random fashion and instead begin to gain confidence in your ability to answer the questions utilizing the four phase process. An answer key, which is located at the conclusion of the exercise, indicates the best answer, question type, and content category for each of the sample questions.

1. Therapists routinely assess the amount of assistance a client needs to complete a selected activity. Categories of assistance include maximal, moderate, minimal, stand-by or supervision. This type of classification system is an example of a/an _____ measurement scale?

    1. interval
    2. nominal
    3. ordinal
    4. ratio

2. Chest percussion and vibration are appropriate bronchial drainage techniques for all of the following except the _____?

    1. anterior apical segment
    2. lingula
    3. left middle lobe
    4. right middle lobe

3. A client diagnosed with chondromalacia patellae is referred to physical therapy. During the initial examination, the therapist measures the client's Q angle as 23 degrees bilaterally. Which clinical finding is not typically associated with an increased Q angle?

    1. increased lateral tibial torsion
    2. genu valgum
    3. increased femoral anteversion
    4. patella alta

4. A client seen twice in physical therapy calls her therapist and states that she is no longer interested in therapy and will not return for any additional appointments. The therapist inquires as to the reason for this decision, but the client refuses to provide any additional information. The therapist's most immediate response should be to _____?

    1. inform the referring physician of the client's decision
    2. document the incident in the medical record
    3. call back and ask the client to reschedule
    4. notify the insurance company of the client's decision

5. A therapist designs a treatment program for a client with a nasogastric tube. Which of the following activities should be avoided when treating the client?

   1. ambulatory distances greater than 100 feet
   2. forward bending range of motion exercises of the head and neck
   3. static balance activities in sitting
   4. shoulder flexion and extension resistive exercises

6. A therapist performs passive range of motion to the lower extremities of a client in the medical intensive care unit. While treating the client, an alarm on one of the monitoring devices sounds. If the therapist is unfamiliar with the particular piece of monitoring equipment, his most immediate response should be to _____?

   1. contact the client's referring physician
   2. contact a member of the nursing staff
   3. attempt to locate a switch to disable the monitoring equipment
   4. disregard the alarm and continue with treatment

7. A therapist designs an exercise program for a client with peripheral vascular disease. The client has decreased peripheral pulses and cool skin, however does not exhibit any signs of resting claudication. Which of the following exercise parameters would be the most beneficial for the client?

   1. short intervals of low level exercise
   2. short intervals of high level exercise
   3. long intervals of low level exercise
   4. long intervals of high level exercise

8. A therapist assesses wrist radial and ulnar deviation with a goniometer. When measuring radial and ulnar deviation, the therapist should position the axis of the goniometer most closely to which carpal bone?

   1. capitate
   2. lunate
   3. trapezium
   4. trapezoid

9. Individual health care organizations have the responsibility to safeguard their clients' medical records. Which of the following situations would require prior consent for the use of a client's medical records?

   1. financial audits
   2. quality assurance
   3. transfer of records to another health care organization
   4. research where anonymity is preserved

10. While ambulating with an above knee prosthesis, a client demonstrates an abducted gait on the prosthetic side. Which of the following is least likely to cause this type of gait deviation?

1. tightness of the gluteus medius
2. discomfort on the adductor longus tendon
3. the medial wall of the prosthesis is too low
4. the prosthetic limb is too long

Answer Key

1. Answer: 3   Resource: Best (146)
   Question Type: What/Which
   Content Area: Intervention

   An ordinal scale permits the ranking of items, however the actual difference between adjacent ranks may not be equal.

2. Answer: 3   Resource: Brannon (43)
   Question Type: What/Which
   Content Area: Intervention

   The left lung does not have a middle lobe.

3. Answer: 4   Resource: Magee (567)
   Question Type: What/Which
   Content Area: Assessment and Evaluation

   Research indicates that a Q angle of less than 13 degrees is often associated with patella alta.

4. Answer: 2   Resource: Kettenbach (31)
   Question Type: How/When
   Content Area: Intervention

   It is necessary for the therapist to document the phone conversation in the medical record in a timely fashion.

5. Answer: 2   Resource: Pierson (265)
   Question Type: How/When
   Content Area: Interpretation and Planning

   A nasogastric tube is a plastic device that is inserted through the nostril and into the stomach. Movements of the head and neck can be disruptive.

6. Answer: 2   Resource: Guide for Professional
   Question Type: How/When   Conduct
   Content Area: Intervention

   Since the therapist is unfamiliar with the monitoring device it is necessary to contact
   another health care professional. The most accessible and logical choice would be
   a member of the nursing staff.

7. Answer: 3   Resource: Brannon (374)
   Question Type: Why
   Content Area: Interpretation and Planning

   The treatment objective for clients with peripheral vascular disease is to increase
   peripheral circulation, therefore, the most beneficial exercise parameter is long
   intervals of low level exercise.

8. Answer: 1   Resource: Norkin and White (88)
   Question Type: Where
   Content Area: Assessment and Evaluation

   When measuring radial and ulnar deviation the axis of the goniometer is placed over
   the middle of the dorsal aspect of the wrist over the capitate.

9. Answer: 3   Resource: Scott - Promoting Legal
   Question Type: What/Which   Awareness (118)
   Content Area: Intervention

   Failure to obtain informed consent from a client prior to releasing medical records
   can be considered healthcare malpractice.

10. Answer: 3   Resource: O'Sullivan (415)
    Question Type: Why
    Content Area: Interpretation and Planning

    A low medial wall would not cause an abducted gait deviation, a high medial wall
    could be a potential cause.

Time Constraints

Like many objective examinations, candidates have a specified amount of time to complete
the Physical Therapist Examination. For physical therapists, the available time is four
hours. Since the examination consists of 200 questions, candidates will have 72 seconds
available to answer each question. This number, although correct when viewing the
examination as a whole, can be misleading. There will be many questions which a
candidate will be able to answer in much less than 72 seconds, whereas other questions
will take somewhat longer. The key to success lies in progressing through the examination
in a consistent and predictable manner.

Although 72 seconds per question does not seem like a great deal of time, the majority of
candidates will have ample time to complete the examination. Despite this fact, it is

important to pay attention to the elapsed time during the examination. It also is important to know your test taking history. Are you typically one of the first, one of the last, or somewhere in the middle of individuals completing an examination? This information is important as you plan your test taking strategy. Regardless of where you fall on the time spectrum, it is important not to be influenced by individuals who complete the examination rapidly.

In order to make sure your pace is appropriate, we suggest placing a small notation in the margin next to question number 50, 100, 150, and 200. If you are taking the actual Physical Therapist Examination, the same objective can be accomplished by writing the question numbers on a piece of paper and placing it next to the computer. These notations should remind candidates to check on the elapsed time at selected intervals throughout the examination. This technique will allow candidates to assess their progress and modify their pace, if needed. Specific guidelines are difficult to determine; however, in general candidates should answer a minimum of 50 questions an hour.

Exercise

Candidates will have 60 minutes to complete the following 50 question examination. The allotted time is consistent with the available time per question on the Physical Therapist Examination. Set a timer for 60 minutes and begin the sample examination. Candidates should use the four phase process as they progress through the examination. An answer key is located at the conclusion of the exercise.

1. A therapist passively moves a client's upper extremity through a selected range of motion while the client's eyes are closed. The client then is asked to verbally describe the direction and range of movement of the upper extremity. This technique can be used to examine _____?

    1. barognosis
    2. graphesthesia
    3. kinesthesia
    4. stereognosis

2. A 16 year old basketball player is anxious to return to athletic competition following rehabilitation from an achilles tendon rupture. The athlete is objectively ready to return to competition; however continues to demonstrate a severe preoccupation with reinjury. The most appropriate response is to _____?

    1. allow the client to return to basketball without restriction
    2. inform the client that he should not participate in basketball this season
    3. design a functional progression for basketball which allows the client to progress to higher level activities in a gradual fashion
    4. discuss other less demanding athletic activities with the client

3. A client with latissimus dorsi and lower trapezius weakness would have the most difficulty performing which of the following activities?

    1. four point gait with Lofstrand crutches
    2. three point gait with a straight cane
    3. swing through gait with crutches
    4. wheelchair propulsion

4. A physical therapist records the vital signs of a 42 year old male before beginning an exercise program. The therapist determines that the client's respiration rate and pulse rate are within normal ranges. If the therapist expresses the value as a ratio of respiratory rate to pulse rate, which of the following would be considered normal?

    1. 1:5
    2. 1:3
    3. 4:1
    4. 6:1

5. A therapist identifies several inconsistencies between a client's subjective complaints and the objective findings of an initial examination. A detailed discussion of the identified inconsistencies belongs in the _____ section of a SOAP note?

    1. subjective
    2. objective
    3. assessment
    4. plan

6. A client eight days status post right total hip replacement loses his balance and falls to the ground. The client is visibly shaken by the fall, but insists that he is uninjured. The therapist examines the right hip and although active motion elicits pain, all other findings are inconclusive. The therapist should immediately _____?

    1. continue with the current treatment so the client does not focus on the incident
    2. notify the director of rehabilitation about the incident
    3. document the incident and contact a physician to examine the client
    4. document the incident and gradually resume prior treatment

7. A 21 year old male suffers a primary dislocation of his right shoulder playing football. The athlete is referred to physical therapy after three weeks of immobilization. A therapist might elect to begin treatment with all of the following except _____?

    1. isometric shoulder exercises
    2. passive range of motion exercises
    3. active assistive range of motion exercises
    4. high speed isokinetic exercises

8. A therapist completes an upper extremity goniometric examination. The therapist records right active elbow range of motion as 15 - 0 - 150 degrees. The total available elbow range of motion for this client is _____ degrees?

    1. 135
    2. 150
    3. 165
    4. 180

9. A therapist conducts a study which measures knee flexion range of motion two weeks following arthroscopic surgery. Assuming a normal distribution, what percentage of clients participating in the study would you expect to achieve a goniometric measurement value greater than one standard deviation below the mean?

    1. 49%
    2. 64%
    3. 68%
    4. 84%

10. A therapist examines a client with unilateral lower extremity weakness. As the client performs hip flexion in supine the therapist helps the client complete the full range of motion. This would best be described as _____?

    1. active exercise
    2. passive exercise
    3. resistive exercise
    4. active-assistive exercise

11. A client recovering from a traumatic brain injury is screened for inclusion in a formal rehabilitation program. Which of the following situations would most prohibit the client from being involved in the rehabilitation program?

    1. inability to sit supported for 60 minutes
    2. inability to tolerate intense rehabilitation
    3. maximal assistance is required with all transfers
    4. failure to be medically stable

12. A therapist completes ambulation activities with a client rehabilitating from a total hip replacement. Later while documenting in the medical record, the therapist realizes she has exceeded the client's prescribed weightbearing status. The most immediate therapist action is to _____?

    1. disregard the incident
    2. discuss the situation with the director of rehabilitation
    3. inform the orthopedic surgeon of the incident
    4. complete an incident report

13. A client is unable to actively participate during a transfer and as a result requires a two man lift to be moved into bed. The most appropriate documentation of transfer status is _____?

   1. the client requires maximal assistance for transfers
   2. the client requires maximal assist of two for transfers
   3. the client is dependent requiring a two man lift transfer
   4. the client requires moderate assist in a two man lift transfer

14. A therapist examines a client status post stroke at bedside. The client is unable to move without assistance. The therapist's highest priority should be _____?

   1. toilet transfers
   2. positioning
   3. gait analysis
   4. cognitive assessment

15. A client two weeks status post CVA has increasing hypertonicity in his hemiplegic upper extremity. All of the following would be indicated as treatment except _____?

   1. use of a sling
   2. active assistive exercise
   3. passive range of motion
   4. weightbearing techniques

16. A client with chronic venous insufficiency presents with significant edema in both lower extremities. Which treatment option would be the most appropriate for the initial visit?

   1. intermittent compression and client education
   2. custom fitted stockings
   3. intermittent compression and warm whirlpool
   4. instruction in a lower extremity exercise program

17. A physical therapist completes a research study that examines the relationship between elbow position and grip strength. The most important action to benefit the field of physical therapy is to _____?

   1. describe the design procedures in sufficient detail
   2. disseminate the results of the research study
   3. develop additional ideas for future research
   4. identify how the research study relates to the current body of knowledge

18. A client recently involved in a motor vehicle accident is referred to physical therapy after being diagnosed with a cervical strain. During the examination the therapist palpates the anterior aspect of the neck. Which of the following bony structures is most superior?

    1. thyroid cartilage
    2. first cricoid ring
    3. hyoid bone
    4. C5 vertebral body

19. A client rehabilitating from a fractured humerus develops a resultant musculocutaneous nerve lesion. Which objective finding is most indicative of musculocutaneous nerve involvement?

    1. weakness of shoulder medial rotation
    2. sensory loss in the lateral forearm
    3. winging of the inferior angle of the scapula
    4. loss of contour in the shoulder due to deltoid paralysis

20. A client diagnosed with Erb-Duchenne paralysis is referred to physical therapy. The medical record indicates the client sustained the injury at birth. Which of the following objective findings would not be expected based on the client's diagnosis?

    1. paralysis of the biceps and brachialis
    2. absent sensation in the deltoid region
    3. absent biceps and brachioradialis reflex
    4. paralysis of the intrinsic hand muscles

21. A therapist completes a series of resisted tests on a client referred to physical therapy with a lower extremity injury. During the testing the client indicates that he begins to experience pain after a number of repetitions. The most likely explanation is _____?

    1. a complete tendon rupture
    2. capsular laxity
    3. intermittent claudication
    4. emotional hypersensitivity

22. A clinical instructor demonstrates a mobilization technique for a student. The clinical instructor describes the movement as a large amplitude movement that does not reach the limit of the range. This description is most representative of _____?

    1. grade I
    2. grade II
    3. grade III
    4. grade IV

23. An administrator in a rehabilitation hospital presents an inservice on legal and ethical issues for health care practitioners. During the inservice the administrator reviews several types of law that affect the health care system. Which type of law is based on court judgments, decisions, and decrees?

    1. constitutional law
    2. statutory law
    3. common law
    4. administrative law

24. A therapist examines a client's sputum sample. The therapist describes the color of the sample as yellow. Which condition is most likely associated with a yellow sputum sample?

    1. pulmonary edema
    2. neoplasm
    3. infection
    4. pneumonia

25. A client diagnosed with peripheral vascular disease is examined in physical therapy. Which of the following objective findings would result in exercise being contraindicated?

    1. decreased peripheral pulses
    2. resting claudication
    3. increased resting systolic blood pressure
    4. decreased lower extremity strength

26. A therapist observes that a number of physical therapy aides often jeopardize client safety when performing selected transfers. The most immediate intervention is to _____?

    1. offer to assist physical therapy aides with selected transfers
    2. prohibit physical therapy aides from performing selected transfers
    3. develop a formal training session on appropriate transfer techniques
    4. provide written literature which outlines basic transfer techniques

27. A client rehabilitating from a motor vehicle accident complains that his pain medication is overdue. The most appropriate therapist action is to _____?

    1. administer the client's pain medication
    2. ask the client to focus on the treatment session and not the pain
    3. notify the nursing staff of the client's complaint
    4. document the client's complaint in the medical record

28. A 63 year old male is referred to physical therapy after being diagnosed with Parkinson's disease. Which of the following should be given the highest priority during the initial treatment session?

1. introducing the client to other client's with Parkinson's disease
2. determining the client's educational background and general knowledge
3. explaining to the client the role of the physical therapist
4. determining the client's current functional status

29. A client in an acute care hospital attempts to get out of bed in preparation for ambulation activities. The client has not been able to ambulate since being admitted to the hospital four weeks ago. The most immediate therapist action is to _____?

1. disconnect the client's intravenous line
2. provide a straight cane for ambulation activities
3. have the client sit on the edge of the bed with his feet on the floor
4. instruct family members in various transfer techniques

30. A therapist performs daily goniometric measurements on a client status post total knee arthroplasty. To ensure the most reliable goniometric measurement, the therapist should _____?

1. utilize the same goniometer for each measurement
2. accurately identify appropriate bony landmarks
3. perform goniometric measurements at the same time each day
4. provide the client with concise and explicit verbal instructions

31. A therapist attempts to assess the chest mobility of a client diagnosed with chronic obstructive pulmonary disease. To assess lower lobe expansion the therapist should _____?

1. place the tips of the thumbs along the manubrium and extend the fingers laterally around the ribs
2. place the tips of the thumbs at the midsternal line at the sternal notch and extend the fingers above the clavicles
3. place the tips of the thumbs at the xiphoid process and extend the fingers laterally around the ribs
4. place the tips of the thumbs along the client's back at the spinous processes of T10 - T12 and extend the fingers around the ribs

32. A client rehabilitating from a stroke exhibits signs and symptoms of depression. Which of the following is not representative of a client with depression?

1. the client develops unrealistic rehabilitation goals
2. the client exhibits decreased participation in physical therapy
3. the client expresses feelings of worthlessness
4. the client exhibits periods of agitation and loss of energy

33. A therapist completes an examination on a client referred to physical therapy with a cervical strain. During the examination the therapist begins to suspect there may be a lesion interfering with neural conduction. Which resisted test would supply the therapist with information on the C4 myotome?

    1. elbow extension
    2. shoulder abduction
    3. shoulder shrug
    4. elbow flexion

34. A client is referred to physical therapy with a diagnosis of CVA, right hemiplegia. The client's past medical history indicates that the client's left knee does not flex past 80 degrees secondary to an accident 20 years ago. The client's home has multiple one step doorways in which the height is 8 inches. Presently the client is unable to descend stairs with the right leg first due to limited left knee range of motion. The most appropriate course of action is to _____?

    1. perform step training using the left leg first when descending
    2. perform step training with the right leg first in an attempt to increase left knee range of motion
    3. discontinue step training until the left knee can flex to 90-100 degrees
    4. consider a temporary ramp until the client can descend stairs properly

35. A therapist attempts to identify an appropriate statistical test to analyze a set of data. In order to use a parametric test, the data should be of a/an _____ level of measurement?

    1. nominal or ordinal
    2. ordinal or interval
    3. nominal or interval
    4. interval or ratio

36. A 72 year old male status post stroke is referred to physical therapy. The client is able to ambulate independently and has good upper extremity strength, however is unable to communicate through verbal or written means. This type of deficit is best termed _____?

    1. apraxia
    2. aphasia
    3. aphonia
    4. aplasia

37. As part of a quality assurance program, a physical therapy department embarks on an outcome assessment study. When working with outcome assessment the most critical period of time is _____?

    1. at the conclusion of a selected treatment session
    2. at the conclusion of care in relation to the goals of treatment
    3. at the conclusion of a 14 day period
    4. after a scheduled physician visit

38. A client is diagnosed with a bacteriocidal infection shortly after being admitted to the hospital. Which of the following laboratory tests would you expect to be most affected based on the client's diagnosis?

    1. platelet count
    2. hemoglobin
    3. hematocrit
    4. white blood cell count

39. A therapist examines a client referred to physical therapy with low back pain. During the examination the therapist determines that the client is restricted in a capsular pattern at the hip. Which of the following motions would you expect to be most limited at the hip?

    1. flexion and extension
    2. abduction and medial rotation + flexion
    3. adduction and lateral rotation
    4. abduction and extension

40. A client scheduled to undergo thoracic surgery is given preoperative instructions. During the training session the client seems very discouraged and anxious about the impending surgery. The most appropriate mechanism to offer emotional support is to _____?

    1. tell the client he will do just fine
    2. notify family members of the client's present state
    3. visit the client immediately after surgery
    4. listen to the client express his feelings

41. A client diagnosed with chronic venous insufficiency is referred to physical therapy. After evaluating the client, the therapist's general treatment goal is to increase venous return and reduce edema. Which of the following would not be part of the expected plan of care?

    1. manual massage of the extremities in a proximal to distal direction
    2. use of an intermittent compression pump
    3. avoid prolonged periods of static standing and sitting with legs dependent
    4. elevation of the foot of the bed during rest

42. A therapist assists a client rehabilitating from shoulder surgery with Codman's pendulum exercises. While performing the exercises the client begins to experience back pain. The most appropriate modified client position would be _____?

    1. supine
    2. standing
    3. sidelying
    4. prone

43. A therapist teaches a client with limited shoulder range of motion a self-mobilization technique. The therapist instructs the client to sit on a firm table and grasp his fingers under the edge of the table. The client is then asked to lean his trunk away from the stabilized arm. This type of self-mobilization technique can be used to facilitate _____?

    1. flexion
    2. internal rotation
    3. external rotation
    4. abduction

    Caudal glide = abduction

44. A 65 year old female rehabilitating from a motor vehicle accident is referred to therapy for treatment of lymphedema. Which of the following would not be part of the expected plan of care?

    1. application of local heat
    2. isometric and isotonic pumping exercises of the distal muscles
    3. elevation of the extremity above the level of the heart
    4. intermittent mechanical compression

45. A therapist examines a 55 year old male whose subjective complaints include asymmetric pain in the knees and hips. The client describes the intensity of the pain in proportion to the amount of daily activity. The client indicates he has been employed as a roofer for the past 20 years. Which disease category is most consistent with this case?

    1. systemic lupus erythematosus
    2. osteoarthritis
    3. rheumatoid arthritis
    4. gout

46. A team of health care professionals develop a rehabilitation management program for a client recovering from a traumatic brain injury. Which of the following steps would be the last to occur?

    1. develop long term rehabilitation goals with the client and family
    2. develop short term goals and treatment priorities
    3. identify significant impairments and disabilities
    4. identify tasks and activities that the client expects to resume

47. A therapist administers the Fugl-Meyer to clients status post stroke in an attempt to identify individuals that may benefit from inclusion in a formal rehabilitation program. What is the primary weakness of this standardized instrument?

    1. poor sensitivity
    2. time consuming
    3. low sensitivity
    4. poor theoretical rationale

48. A therapist screens a client status post stroke for placement in a formal rehabilitation program. The client is medically stable, however needs 24 hour per day monitoring and moderate assistance with mobility and activities of daily living. The client is presently able to tolerate intense rehabilitation three hours per day. The most appropriate setting for continued therapy is _____?

    1. an inpatient rehabilitation hospital
    2. a nursing facility
    3. home care
    4. an acute care hospital

49. A client diagnosed with a grade I anterior talofibular ligament sprain is referred to physical therapy. The best indicator of the client's expected functional status following rehabilitation would be based on _____?

    1. the client's previous functional status
    2. the number of physical therapy visits
    3. the quality of the physical therapy services
    4. the client's willingness to complete a home exercise program

50. A client rehabilitating from congestive heart failure is examined in physical therapy. During the examination the client begins to complain of pain. The most appropriate therapist action is to _____?

    1. notify the nursing staff to administer pain medication
    2. contact the referring physician
    3. discontinue the treatment session
    4. ask the client to describe the location and severity of the pain

Answer Key

1. Answer: 3   Resource: Thomas (1053)

   Kinesthesia is defined as the ability to perceive extent, direction or weight of movement.

2. Answer: 3   Resource: Booher (236)

   The treatment plan should allow the client to gradually gain confidence in his ability to return to athletic competition while at the same time have the opportunity to perform sport specific skills.

3. Answer: 3   Resource: Minor (299)

   A swing through gait pattern with crutches requires significant upper extremity strength and scapular stability. It is often used with clients who have lower extremity weakness or paralysis.

4. Answer: 1   Resource: Minor (39)

   Although normal values deviate from source to source, broad ranges of normal values for heart rate and respiration rate are as follows: Heart rate 60-100 beats per minute, respiration rate 12-18 breaths/minute.

5. Answer: 3   Resource: Kettenbach (110)

   The assessment section of a SOAP note provides a platform for a therapist to express his/her professional judgment.

6. Answer: 3   Resource: Guide for Professional Conduct

   Since the therapist's findings were inconclusive and the client is status post total hip replacement it is necessary for the client to be examined by a physician.

7. Answer: 4   Resource: Kisner (303)

   High speed isokinetic exercises would be an inappropriate treatment option based on the client's current status.

8. Answer: 3   Resource: Norkin and White (26)

   Since the 15 is to the left of 0 it is indicative of hyperextension, therefore 150 + 15 = 165.

9. Answer: 4   Resource: Best (221)

A normal distribution produces a bell shaped curve where predictable percentages of the population can be determined. 50% of the population falls on each side of the mean and 34% of the population falls between -1 standard deviation and the mean (50% +34% = 84%).

10. Answer: 4   Resource: Minor (134)

Active assisted exercise requires movement performed by a client with additional movement or mechanical assistance.

11. Answer: 4   Resource: Post-Stroke
                                                         Rehabilitation (73)

A formal rehabilitation program often requires a minimum of 3 hours of services from physical therapy, occupational therapy and speech. Failure to be medically stable would prohibit this type of participation.

12. Answer: 4   Resource: Scott - Promoting Legal
                                                         Awareness (69)

An incident report should be completed which will serve to provide details of the event in question.

13. Answer: 3   Resource: Kettenbach (49)

The most appropriate form of documentation describes the type of transfer and the amount of assistance necessary to complete the transfer.

14. Answer: 2   Resource: Minor (116)

Positioning should be the therapist's highest priority in order to avoid contractures and tissue breakdown.

15. Answer: 1   Resource: Davies (212)

The use of a sling is not indicated in the treatment of hypertonicity since it will serve to immobilize the arm and reinforce a flexor synergy pattern.

16. Answer: 1   Resource: Kisner (638)

The primary goal of treatment is to increase venous return and reduce edema. Intermittent compression will assist with this goal and client education will be directed toward decreasing dependent edema.

17. Answer: 2   Resource: Currier (321)

Disseminating the results of a research study is the primary means of expanding the professions body of knowledge.

18. Answer: 3   Resource: Hoppenfeld (106)

The hyoid bone is located at the same level as the C3 vertebral body. The thyroid cartilage is directly below the hyoid bone.

19. Answer: 2   Resource: Magee (223)

In addition to sensory loss in the lateral forearm an injury to the musculocutaneous nerve can result in loss of elbow flexion, shoulder forward flexion and decreased supination.

20. Answer: 4   Resource: Pauls (413)

The intrinsic muscles of the hand are primarily innervated by nerve roots C8-T1. Erb-Duchenne palsy is an upper brachial plexus injury typically involving the roots of C5-C6.

21. Answer: 3   Resource: Kisner (631)

Insufficient blood supply to an exercising muscle or group of muscles can result in intermittent claudication.

22. Answer: 2   Resource: Kisner (194)

Grade II oscillations are defined as large amplitude within the range, not reaching the limit.

23. Answer: 3   Resource: Scott - Promoting Legal Awareness (5)

Common law develops over time based on judicial decisions. It is also referred to as judge-made case law.

24. Answer: 3   Resource: Rothstein (533)

Yellow or greenish sputum is commonly associated with acute or chronic infection.

25. Answer: 2   Resource: Kisner (636)

Clients with peripheral vascular disease that present with resting claudication are not considered candidates for exercise.

26. Answer: 2   Resource: Standards of Practice

The physical therapy aides should not be permitted to perform transfers until a remediation plan is developed and implemented.

27. Answer: 3   Resource: Guide for Professional Conduct

The nursing staff is the appropriate party to assess the veracity of the clients complaint and if necessary administer the pain medication.

28. Answer: 4   Resource: O'Sullivan (479)

By assessing the clients functional status the therapist will be able to gain valuable information necessary to design a comprehensive plan of care. It will also provide the therapist with a means to assess the future performance of the client.

29. Answer: 3   Resource: Miller-Keane (792)

Since the client has been a significant amount of time without ambulating it is advisable to assist him/her to a standing position in a gradual fashion. This will help to avoid the client feeling light headed, dizzy or exhibiting signs of postural hypotension.

30. Answer: 2   Resource: Norkin and White (35)

Although each of the options has an influence on the reliability of goniometric measurements, identifying the appropriate bony landmarks is fundamental to any goniometric measurement.

31. Answer: 4   Resource: Irwin (342)

The examination procedure allows the therapist to compare the timing and degree of movement of each hand during quiet and deep breathing.

32. Answer: 1   Resource: Miller-Keane (431)

Depression is defined as a morbid sadness, dejection, or melancholy, distinguished from grief, which is realistic and proportionate to a personal loss.

33. Answer: 3   Resource: Kendall (282)

The trapezius is innervated by the spinal portion of cranial nerve XI and ventral ramus of C2, C3, and C4. The upper trapezius assists with the ability to approximate the acromion and occiput.

34. Answer: 1   Resource: Minor (308)

Although not the preferred method, by descending with the left knee first the client may be able to safely and efficiently travel through the one step doorways.

35. Answer: 4   Resource: Best (207)

Parametric tests assume that data is normally or near normally distributed. Parametric tests are applied to both interval and ratio data.

36. Answer: 2   Resource: Miller-Keane (116)

Aphasia is defined as the loss of power of expression by speech, writing, or signs due to disease or injury of the brain center.

37. Answer: 2   Resource: Walter (244)

Outcome assessment studies tend to compare a client's status at the time of discharge in relation to the expected goals of treatment.

38. Answer: 4   Resource: Goodman (456)

Lymphocytes, monocytes and granulocytes are types of white blood cells encountered with infection.

39. Answer: 2   Resource: Magee (460)

A capsular pattern of restriction at the hip includes flexion, abduction, and medial rotation.

40. Answer: 4   Resource: Davis (101)

Listening to the client express his/her feelings demonstrates respect for his/her present emotional state. Actions to dismiss the client's feelings are insensitive and can damage the client-therapist relationship.

41. Answer: 1   Resource: Kisner (639)

Massage techniques utilized on a client with chronic venous insufficiency should be in a distal to proximal direction.

42. Answer: 4   Resource: Kisner (282)

Codman's pendulum exercises can be performed with the client in prone on a plinth with the arm over the side. It is not as desirable as a standing position since it is difficult to initiate movement using the trunk in the prone position.

43. Answer: 4   Resource: Kisner (284)

This type of self-mobilization activity produces a caudal glide which is used to increase abduction of the glenohumeral joint.

44. Answer: 1   Resource: Kisner (641)

Application of local heat will place an increased demand on the lymphatic system and should therefore be avoided.

45. Answer: 2   Resource: Pauls (82)

Osteoarthritis is a chronic degenerative disorder that leads to the breakdown of the articular cartilage of synovial joints. Joints most commonly affected are the weight bearing joints. Pain is typically worse with activity and morning stiffness is often present.

46. Answer: 2   Resource: Kettenbach (97)

Short term goals are building blocks which often identify treatment priorities and provide a platform for the achievement of an associated long term goal.

47. Answer: 2   Resource: Post-Stroke
                                                   Rehabilitation (232)

Fugl-Meyer scale of functional return after hemiplegia assesses items such as muscle tone, state of motor recovery, synergy, movement speed and prehension pattern of the limbs. The Fugl-Meyer can take in excess of 20 minutes to complete, however has been shown to be reliable and valid in clients with hemiplegia.

48. Answer: 1   Resource: Post-Stroke
                                                   Rehabilitation (73)

Medically stable clients able to tolerate intense rehabilitation for three hours per day are often good candidates for rehabilitation. 24 hour per day monitoring and assistance with mobility and activities of daily living are available at inpatient rehabilitation hospitals.

49. Answer: 1   Resource: Kisner (484)

A grade I ligament sprain is a relatively minor injury that is often resolved in 1-2 weeks. As a result, the client's previous functional status should serve as an ideal predictor of functional status following rehabilitation.

50. Answer: 4   Resource: Magee (3)

Although a subjective report of pain is relevant information, additional information must be gathered prior to determining its significance.

This activity should have provided candidates with a basic understanding of the time available to answer a selected number of questions. Candidates should, however, recognize that taking a 50 question examination in 60 minutes is much different than taking the actual Physical Therapist Examination. Issues such as the environment, concentration, and endurance, which for most candidates are not relevant when taking a 50 question examination, can be very relevant when candidates are subjected to the actual examination.

The most effective way to determine if the time constraints of the Physical Therapist Examination will affect you is to practice taking 200 question sample examinations. This activity will not only reduce your anxiety level about the time constraints, but will also allow you to make changes in your pace, if necessary, prior to the actual examination.

Unit Eight contains a 200 question sample examination. Additional information on review books and computer software designed for the Physical Therapist Examination is located at the conclusion of the text.

Unit Six
Content Outline

Perhaps the most valuable piece of information a candidate can utilize when preparing for the Physical Therapist Examination is the content outline. The content outline provides a detailed analysis of each of the three content areas of the Physical Therapist Examination. A thorough understanding of each of the content areas and the corresponding subtopics will streamline a candidate's preparation. Less time will be spent covering topics that are not clinically relevant to the actual examination and as a result, more time will be available for reviewing and relearning.

The chart below illustrates the three content areas of the Physical Therapist Examination and the percentage of examination items in each content area.

Physical Therapist Examination

Content Outline

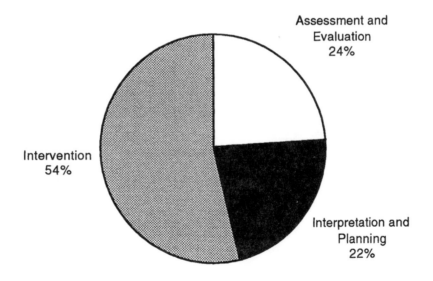

The actual number of questions in each content area for the 200 question Physical Therapist Examination can be determined based on the given percentage of examination items. The following table identifies the number of questions in each of the three content areas on the Physical Therapist Examination.

Content Areas	Number of Questions
Assessment and Evaluation	48
Interpretation and Planning	44
Intervention	108
	Total = 200

Exercise

The following exercise will explore the content outline in greater detail. Individual subtopics in each content area will be analyzed. A brief general statement regarding the subject matter in each subtopic is presented along with an outline of associated information.

Five sample questions will be presented for candidates to answer in each subtopic. Candidates should recognize that these questions represent only a small fraction of the potential questions that could appear on the actual examination. Additional sample questions for each of the subtopics will appear in the sample examination contained in Unit Eight. Candidates should use this exercise not only to become familiar with the content outline, but also to refine their test taking skills.

Attempt to identify the best answer to each of the 50 questions and mark the answer in the appropriate space on the enclosed answer sheet. After completing the exercise, utilize the answer key located at the conclusion of the exercise to determine the number of questions answered correctly.

Physical Therapist Examination

Content Outline Analysis

I. Assessment and Evaluation

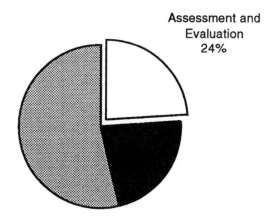

Assessment and
Evaluation
24%

Assessment and Evaluation	Number of Questions
General Procedures	
Data Collection	14
Test/Measurements	22
System Specific Procedures	12
	Total = 48

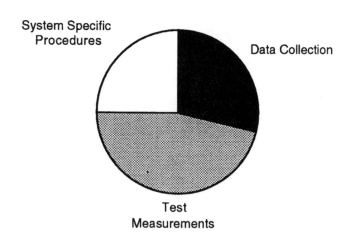

System Specific
Procedures

Data Collection

Test
Measurements

75

A. General Procedures

1. Data Collection

Data collection is an essential aspect of a standard client assessment. The collected information provides the foundation on which to construct an appropriate client care plan. Therapists utilize resources such as the client interview and the medical record to obtain necessary information.

Client Medical Record	Diagnosis
Physician Referral	Results of Diagnostic Testing
Laboratory Results	Client History
Age	Mechanism and Date of Injury
Chief Complaint	Aggravating/Relieving Factors
Knowledge of Condition	Goals and Expectations
Functional Status	Premorbid Lifestyle
Occupation	Medications
Restrictions/Precautions	Social History
Psychosocial History	Family Medical History
Observation	Inspection
Environment	Identify Available Resources
Professional Consultation	

Sample Questions

1. While obtaining a client history, it is important not to ask leading questions, which may elicit irrelevant or inaccurate information. Which of the following questions might be considered the most leading?

    1. Where is your pain located?
    2. When did the present pain arise?
    3. Which activities are particularly difficult to perform?
    4. Do you have pain in the morning?

2. A therapist interviews a 21 year old football player referred to physical therapy after sustaining a grade II acromioclavicular sprain. Which of the following client descriptions best describes the injury mechanism associated with an acromioclavicular sprain?

    1. "I was being tackled and landed directly on my shoulder."
    2. "I fell with my arm extended and another player fell on top of me."
    3. "My arm was hit with a helmet while I was throwing the ball."
    4. "My arm was stepped on while I was laying on the ground."

3. A client diagnosed with an anterior cruciate ligament injury is examined in physical therapy. During the examination, the client asks the therapist why the physician would order x-rays after already diagnosing the ligament injury. The primary purpose for ordering the radiographs would be to _____?

   1. confirm the physician's diagnosis
   2. check for possible meniscal involvement
   3. examine the client's skeletal maturity
   4. rule out the possibility of a fracture

4. A client diagnosed with impingement syndrome is referred to physical therapy. During the client's initial examination, the therapist identifies several clinical findings that indicate the possibility of a small rotator cuff tear. The therapist's most appropriate action would be to _____?

   1. contact the referring physician to discuss the clinical findings
   2. treat the client as diagnosed on the referral
   3. refer the client back to the physician
   4. discharge the client from physical therapy

5. A self referred client is examined in physical therapy. The therapist asks the client a variety of questions in an attempt to rule out systemic involvement. Which of the following questions would provide the most direct information on the presence of a brain tumor?

   1. Have you had any unusual headaches or changes in your vision?
   2. Can you think of any time during the past week when you may have fallen or been injured?
   3. Have you had any sudden weight loss in the last three weeks without dieting?
   4. Have you noticed any change in your bowel movements or flow of urination?

2. Test/Measurements

Therapists utilize numerous test/measures to obtain objective information during a client assessment. Therapists should select and justify appropriate test/measures for clients based on variables such as medical diagnosis, current status and functional needs. Therapists should be sensitive to issues such as reliability, validity and the sources of error associated with each test/measure.

General Considerations

Purpose	Selection
Precautions	Reliability
Validity	Preparation
Positioning	Implementation
Tolerance	Signs of Physiologic Distress
Modification	Interpretation

Arousal, Mentation and Cognition
Level of Consciousness   Level of Recall
Orientation

Tools
Interview   Questionnaire
Standardized Instruments

Inspection
Body Structure and Alignment   Posture
Skin and Nails   Subcutaneous Soft Tissue

Tools
Plumb Line   Postural Examination Chart

Anthropometric Characteristics
Height   Weight
Girth   Length
Body-Fat Composition

Tools
Tape Measure   Electrical Impedance
Calipers   Underwater Weighing
Volumetrics

Active Movements
Range of Motion   Quality of Movement

Tools
Goniometer   Visual Estimation

Passive Movements
Range of Motion   End Feel

Tools
Goniometer   Visual Estimation

Sensation
Pain   Temperature
Light Touch   Pressure
Kinesthesia   Position Sense
Vibration   Stereognosis
Tactile Localization   Two-Point Discrimination
Barognosis   Graphesthesia

Tools
Pin
Test Tubes
Tuning Fork
Keys, Coins, Pencils etc.

Paper Clip
Cotton
Small Weights

Muscle Strength
Electrophysiologic Tests
Manual Muscle Testing

Functional Muscle Testing
Dynamometry

Tools
Hand-held Dynamometer

Isokinetic Dynamometer

Balance
Static
Weight Shifting
Reactions

Dynamic
Perturbation
Synergies

Tools
Standardized Instruments
Ankle Platform System

Therapeutic Ball

Coordination
Equilibrium Tests
Gross Motor Activities
Speed

Nonequilibrium Tests
Fine Motor Activities
Quality

Tools
Standardized Instruments

Stop Watch

Endurance
Heart Sounds
Voice Sounds
Synergy Patterns
Perceived Exertion

Breath Sounds
Substitution Patterns
Target Heart Rate
Signs of Physiologic Distress

Tools
Stethoscope

Perceived Exertion Scales

Palpation
Skin
Bony Structures

Subcutaneous Soft Tissues

Tools
Gloves (if indicated)

Pain
Behavior   Subjective Measures
Objective Measures

Tools
Interview   Questionnaires
Visual Analog Scales   Symptom Magnification Scales

Gait
Phase   Motion
Cadence   Base of Support
Step Length   Step Time
Stride Length   Stride Time

Tools
Stopwatch   Measuring Tape
Gait Analysis Scales   Functional Ambulation Profiles
Videotape Analysis   Electromyographic Analyses
Weightbearing Scales

Functional Status
Bed Mobility   Transfers
Ambulation   Assistive Devices
Activities of Daily Living   Wheelchair Mobility
Home Assessment   Community Mobility
Recreational Activity

Tools
Stopwatch   Functional Training Scales

Sample Questions

6. A therapist examines a 40 year old female referred to physical therapy after spraining her ankle playing volleyball. During the examination, the client exhibits extreme tenderness to palpation over the sinus tarsi. What ligament is most often associated with tenderness in this area?

    1. anterior talofibular
    2. calcaneofibular
    3. deltoid
    4. posterior talofibular

7. A therapist completes a sensory examination on a client with incomplete T7-T8 paraplegia. The therapist examines the client's sensation using a piece of cotton. The therapist applies the cotton in a random fashion and the client is asked to indicate when she feels the stimulus. This method of sensory testing is used to examine _____?

    1. kinesthesia
    2. light touch
    3. proprioception
    4. superficial pain

8. A physical therapist examines a client who complains of occasional difficulty maintaining her balance when walking and frequent episodes of vertigo. The most likely cause of the client's difficulty is a disorder of the _____ system?

    1. visual
    2. proprioceptive
    3. auditory
    4. vestibular

9. A therapist determines that a client has diminished calf sensation and an absent achilles reflex on the right lower extremity. Earlier the client had communicated to the therapist that she experienced difficulty controlling her bowel movements. The neurologic level of most concern is _____?

    1. L2
    2. L4
    3. L5
    4. S2

10. A therapist determines that a client has a one half inch leg length discrepancy. The therapist suspects the client's leg length discrepancy may be due to tibial shortening. The most appropriate measurement to confirm the therapist's suspicions is from the _____?

    1. anterior superior iliac spine to the medial malleolus
    2. iliac crest to the lateral malleolus
    3. medial knee joint line to the medial malleolus
    4. lateral knee joint line to the medial malleolus

B. System Specific Procedures

Specific procedures exist to assess each system of the body. These procedures are commonly utilized by therapists to collect additional information not obtained using more general procedures. Therapists should be familiar with each of the selected procedures and understand their role in client assessment and examination.

Musculoskeletal Status

Osteokinematics	Arthrokinematics
Accessory Joint Motion	Muscle Tone
Flexibility	Capsular Patterns

Special Tests

Alignment	Joint Dysfunction
Muscle/Tendon Pathology	Muscle Tightness
Ligamentous Instability	Malingering

Tools

Goniometer	Tape Measure

Neuromuscular Status

Deep Tendon Reflexes	Superficial Cutaneous Reflexes
Primitive Reflexes	Clonus

Tools

Reflex Hammer	Large Pin

Cardiopulmonary Status

Blood Pressure	Heart Rate
Respiration Rate	Auscultation
Percussion	Pulses
Chest Mobility	Breathing Patterns
Cough	Sputum
Exercise Testing	Oxygen Saturation

Tools

Stethoscope	Sphygmomanometer
Stopwatch	Support Equipment
Monitoring Equipment	Pulse Oximeter

Integumentary Status

Color	Integrity
Temperature	Moisture
Turgor	Texture
Wound Status	Aseptic Technique

Tools

Measuring Instruments	Protective Equipment

Developmental Status
Developmental Milestones
Cognitive Development
Emotional Development

Physical Development
Social Development

Tools
Standardized Instruments

Sample Questions

11. A therapist examines a client with limited cervical range of motion. As part of the examination, the therapist attempts to screen the client for possible vertebral artery involvement, but is unable to position the client's head and neck in the recommended test position. The most appropriate action is to _____?

    1. complete the vertebral artery test with the head and neck positioned in approximately 50 percent of the available cervical range of motion
    2. complete the vertebral artery test as far into the available cervical range of motion as tolerated
    3. avoid completing the vertebral artery test until the client has full cervical range of motion
    4. avoid all direct cervical treatment techniques until the vertebral artery test can be assessed at the limits of normal cervical range of motion

12. A physical therapist observes the electrocardiogram of a client during exercise. Which of the following ECG changes would be considered abnormal during exercise?

    1. increase in amplitude of P wave
    2. shortening of PR interval
    3. ST segment depression of greater than 1 mm
    4. decrease in amplitude of T wave

13. A therapist positions a client in prone on a plinth and passively flexes her knee. As the knee flexes, the client's hip on the same side also begins to flex. This clinical finding is most indicative of a _____?

    1. tight iliopsoas
    2. tight rectus femoris
    3. tight tensor fasciae latae
    4. tight hamstrings

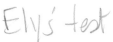
Ely's test

14. A therapist attempts to determine a client's pulse rate immediately after exercise. Which of the following techniques would supply the therapist with the most accurate measurement of pulse rate?

   1.   determine the pulse rate using the brachial artery for 10 seconds and multiply by six
   2.   determine the pulse rate using the femoral artery for 15 seconds and multiply by four
   3.   determine the pulse rate using the radial artery for 30 seconds and multiply by two
   4.   determine the pulse rate using the carotid artery for 60 seconds

15. A therapist assesses a client's lower extremity deep tendon reflexes using a reflex hammer. Which of the following reflexes would provide the therapist with the most information on the L3-L4 neurologic level?

   1.   patellar reflex
   2.   lateral hamstrings reflex
   3.   posterior tibial reflex
   4.   Achilles reflex

II. Interpretation and Planning

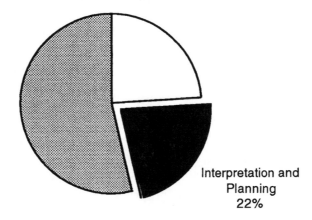

Interpretation and
Planning
22%

Interpretation and Planning	Number of Questions
Data Interpretation	26
Goal Setting and Care Planning	18
Total =	**44**

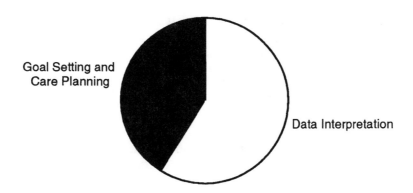

Goal Setting and
Care Planning

Data Interpretation

A. Data Interpretation

Therapists should identify and interpret significant findings from assessment activities. Identification and interpretation of such findings allow therapists to manage their clients' care in an effective and efficient manner.

Normative Values
Extraneous Information
Cause/Effect
Precautions

Essential Information
Problem Identification
Differential Diagnosis
Contraindications

Sample Questions

16. A physical therapist is treating a client with a right transtibial amputation. When ambulating with a patellar-tendon bearing socket, the client complains of discomfort on the patella. The most appropriate treatment to decrease the client's discomfort is to _____?

   1. add a shoe lift to the left leg
   2. add a one ply sock to the residual limb and reapply the prosthesis
   3. discontinue ambulation
   4. place a piece of foam over the patella and reapply the prosthesis

17. A physical therapist begins to gait train a client who recently received an ankle-foot orthosis to assist with foot drop and sensory loss. A reddened area over the lateral malleolus persists after ambulating sixty feet. The most appropriate therapist response is to _____?

   1. direct the client to wear the orthosis at all times because the body will eventually get used to it
   2. direct the client to make an appointment with the orthotist and continue to wear the orthosis until that time
   3. direct the client not to wear the orthosis until modifications are made
   4. direct the client to make an appointment with the physician

18. A client recovering from a serious hamstrings strain is examined isokinetically prior to returning to track competition. Results of the examination reveal peak torque measurements of 125 ft lbs with knee extension and 78 ft lbs with knee flexion at 180 degrees per second on the involved lower extremity. What conclusion can be made regarding the client's ability to return to athletic competition?

   1. The client's quadriceps and hamstrings strength are appropriate for a return to athletic activities.
   2. The client's hamstrings strength demonstrates the need for continued rehabilitation.
   3. The client's quadriceps/hamstrings ratio is below acceptable levels for athletic activities.
   4. Not enough information is given to make an accurate determination of the client's ability to return to athletic competition.

19. A physical therapist receives a referral for a client who is one week status post stroke. When observing the client lying in bed, the therapist notes that the client's calf and foot are edematous. The client reports that the area is somewhat painful. The physical therapist should _____?

    1. discontinue the examination and hope the client's leg is better tomorrow
    2. consider ordering compression stockings for the client
    3. continue with the examination and disregard the client's condition
    4. inform the physician of the situation and discontinue the examination

20. A client in a work hardening program is required to lift packages weighing approximately 30 pounds overhead to a conveyor belt. The client can complete the task, but is unable to prevent excessive lumbar hyperextension while reaching for the conveyor belt. Which of the following assumptions is most accurate?

    1. additional weight should be added to the packages which will promote lumbar stability
    2. the client should continue lifting the 30 pound packages because he will gradually become stronger
    3. the task is too easy for the client
    4. the task is too difficult for the client

B. Goal Setting and Care Planning

Therapists should develop a plan of care for each client based on the results of assessment and examination activities. The established plan of care should be reflective of individual client needs and available resources. Established goals should provide an opportunity to objectively measure client progress.

Goal Setting

Problem List	Long Term Goals
Short Term Goals	Relationship of LTG to STG
Audience	Behavior
Condition	Degree
Prioritization	Clarity
Revision	

Care Planning

Prioritization	Selection
Justification	Treatment Effect
Outcome Measures	Barriers to Client Progress
Discharge Planning	

Sample Questions

21. A therapist examines an 80 year old female four weeks status post stroke. The therapist informs the client that she could benefit from having physical therapy services. The client explains that she is no longer able to drive and is forced to rely on a taxi for all of her transportation. The client further states that the cost of the taxi is prohibitive. The woman resides alone and does not have access to community transport. The most appropriate setting for continued therapy would be _____?

    1. outpatient rehabilitation
    2. skilled nursing facility
    3. home health services
    4. inpatient rehabilitation

22. Which of the following goals is not realistic upon discharge from a phase I cardiac rehabilitation program for a client status post coronary artery bypass graft?

    1. ambulate 100 feet on level surfaces
    2. walk up and down a flight of stairs
    3. locate and recognize changes in pulse rate
    4. range of motion and exercise at 6 METs

23. A client successfully advances through a series of short term goals, but is unable to attain the associated long term goal. The therapist's most appropriate response is to _____?

    1. develop another more attainable long term goal
    2. develop additional short term goals which facilitate achievement of the established long term goal
    3. contact the referring physician to discuss the client's lack of progress
    4. discharge the client since he is no longer making progress toward the established long term goal

24. A client originally referred to physical therapy for six weeks of treatment has achieved all of the established short and long term goals in less than three weeks. The client is completely asymptomatic and has returned to all previously performed activities of daily living. The therapist's most appropriate action is to _____?

    1. continue to treat the client three times a week for the remaining three weeks
    2. reduce the frequency of the client's appointments to twice a week
    3. reduce the frequency of the client's appointments to once a week
    4. discharge the client and send a copy of the discharge summary to the referring physician

25. A physical therapist employed in an acute care hospital returns to work after a brief vacation and finds a number of items that require her immediate attention. Which of the following items should be given the highest priority?

    1.   a message to call a physician
    2.   a client referral from two days ago
    3.   a laboratory test report
    4.   a client record that has not been completed

III. Intervention

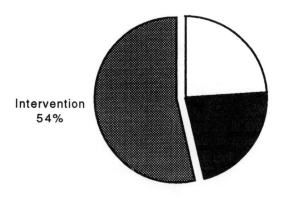

Intervention
54%

Intervention	Number of Questions
Preparation	20
Implementation	46
Education/Communication/Consultation	14
Supporting Activities	16
System Specific Procedures	12
	Total = 108

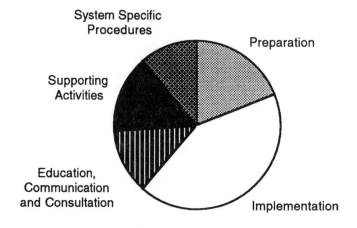

A. Preparation

Therapists need to perform a number of specific activities to prepare for client treatment. These activities are broad in scope and range from inspecting equipment to positioning a client. In all cases, therapists should be aware of safety issues and be responsive to the individual needs of their clients.

Precautions/Contraindications	Obtain Necessary Equipment
Check Equipment Safety	Survey Treatment Area
Positioning	Draping
Privacy	Instruction
Demonstration	Biomechanics
Safety	Work Environment
Ergonomic Design	Accessibility

Sample Questions

26. A home assessment is performed for a client that will utilize a wheelchair. The client's home presently does not possess a ramp and therefore is inaccessible. The distance from the ground to the front doorway is approximately three feet. In order for the client to enter and exit the home safely and independently, the ramp should be at least _____ feet long?

    1. 27
    2. 30
    3. 36
    4. 45

27. A physical therapist examines a 43 year old female diagnosed with a nondisplaced fracture of the humerus. During the examination the client tells the therapist she has kept her arm in a sling sporadically, but would like the therapist's permission to stop using it. An appropriate course of action would be to _____?

    1. instruct the client to wear the sling at all times
    2. instruct the client not to use the sling, because it will inhibit her range of motion
    3. use his/her best judgment based on how the referring physician usually treats humerus fractures
    4. contact the physician and ask what instructions were given to the client

28. A client who is comatose due to a recent head injury receives chest physical therapy. When performing this treatment, the physical therapist should avoid placing the client in _____?

    1. partial sitting using the head of the bed for support
    2. sidelying
    3. Trendelenburg position
    4. semi-prone

29. A physical therapist is treating a client with a diagnosis of chronic arterial insufficiency. Assuming the client does not demonstrate pain at rest, which of the following treatment techniques would be contraindicated for this client?

    1. ambulation with an assistive device
    2. client education regarding proper skin care
    3. stationary cycling
    4. ankle pumps with legs elevated

30. A physical therapy department develops guidelines for electrical equipment care and service. Which of the following guidelines does not meet acceptable equipment care and service standards?

    1. AC power receptacles and plugs should be hospital grade quality
    2. electrical equipment should be inspected every 24-36 months
    3. a file of clinical and technical information for each piece of equipment should be established
    4. documentation of inspection and repair activities should be available for each device

B. Implementation

Therapists should implement appropriate treatment activities for clients with a wide variety of medical conditions. Therapists should utilize available resources to facilitate the achievement of established goals. Selected treatment activities should be individualized to the particular needs of each client and be modified periodically based on reassessment. Therapists should be aware of client response to treatment and be able to offer appropriate intervention when necessary.

Emergency Care Procedures
CPR - Adult/Child/Infant
Emergency Stations
Signs of Distress
Universal Precautions
Autonomic Dysreflexia

First Aid
Codes
Diabetic Conditions
Orthostatic Hypotension
Spinal Shock

Therapeutic Exercise
Stretching
Breathing Exercises
Body Mechanics
Aquatic Exercise
Relaxation Training

Strengthening
Ambulation Training
Leisure Activities
Posture Awareness Training
Home Programs

Therapeutic Modalities/Equipment

Continuous Passive Motion
Tilt Table

Functional Electrical Stimulation

High Voltage Stimulation
Interferential Current
Iontophoresis
Biofeedback
Diathermy
Contrast Bath
Hot Pack
Ultraviolet
Mechanical Traction
Mechanical Compression
Therapeutic Massage
Supportive Equipment

Mechanical Compression
Neuromuscular Electrical
    Stimulation
Transcutaneous Electrical
Nerve Stimulation
Low Voltage Stimulation
Infrared Radiation
Phonophoresis
Ultrasound
Hydrotherapy
Paraffin Bath
Cryotherapy
Hyperbaric Oxygenation
Compression Garments
Fluidotherapy
Monitoring Equipment

Prescribe, Fabricate and/or Apply Assistive and Adaptive Devices

Orthoses
Assistive Devices
Supportive Devices

Prostheses
Adaptive Devices
Protective Devices

Functional Training

Bed Mobility
Ambulation
Wheelchair Management
Recreational Activity
Orthotic/Prosthetic Training
Energy Conservation

Transfers
Activities of Daily Living
Developmental Activity
Assistive/Adaptive Training
Work Simulation

Sample Questions

31. A client that has been on extended bedrest is positioned on a tilt table. After slightly elevating the head of the tilt table, the client begins to demonstrate signs of orthostatic hypotension. The therapist's most immediate response should be to _____?

   1. reassure the client that her response is not unusual
   2. contact the director of rehabilitation for assistance
   3. document the incident in the client's chart
   4. lower the tilt table

32. A therapist receives a referral to instruct a client diagnosed with peroneal tendonitis in a home exercise program. As part of the home exercise program, the therapist would like the client to apply superficial heat to the injured area before beginning a stretching regimen. Which of the following modalities would be the most effective for the client to incorporate into the program?

    1. diathermy
    2. paraffin
    3. pulsed ultrasound
    4. warm water bath

33. A therapist elects to use therapeutic massage on a client diagnosed with a hamstrings strain. The therapist can sense that the client is unsure of what to expect during the massage. The most appropriate massage technique to initiate treatment is _____?

    1. effleurage
    2. petrissage
    3. tapotement
    4. vibration

34. A therapist designs a resistive program utilizing DeLorme and Watkins isotonic training program to strengthen the hamstrings. The program will require the client to complete three sets of 10 repetitions. If the therapist determines the client's ten repetition maximum is eighty pounds, how much weight would the client be instructed to use on the first set?

    1. 20 lbs.
    2. 40 lbs.
    3. 60 lbs.
    4. 80 lbs.

35. A therapist instructs a client how to rise from a chair before beginning ambulation activities with a walker. Which of the following instructions would be helpful to the client?

    1. place both hands on the walker and pull yourself to a standing position
    2. push up on the chair with one hand and place the other hand on the edge of the walker for balance
    3. push up on the chair with both hands and reach for the walker once you are standing
    4. push up on the chair with both hands and reach for the walker while rising

C. Education/Communication/Consultation

Therapists should plan and develop educational programming based on the educational needs of their target audience. They must establish and maintain effective working relationships with other health care personnel and enhance existing lines of communication between colleagues, clients and families. Therapists should maintain objective documentation and indicate progress toward established goals.

Education

Identify Needs	Target Audience
Learning Theory	Domains of Learning
Learning Style	Teaching Strategies
Instruction	Explanation
Media	Resources
Utility of Topic	Objectives
Reinforcement	Feedback
Modification/Revision	Client/Family Education
Staff Education	Community Education
Coping Strategies	Self-Management

Communication

Formal	Informal
Verbal	Written
Medical Record	S.O.A.P. Note
Discharge Summaries	Values
Assertiveness Skills	Chain Of Commands
Rehabilitation Team	

Consultation

Client-related Consultation	Client-related Consultation
Client Rounds	Specialty Care Clinics
Multidisciplinary Meetings	Work Site Analysis
Injury Reduction	Screening
Disease Prevention	American Disabilities Act
Health Promotion	Accessibility
Safety Programs	Policymaking
Expert Legal Opinion	

Sample Questions

36. A physical therapist treats a client with C5-C6 quadriplegia. During the treatment session the client's spouse asks a question regarding the client's ability to transfer independently following rehabilitation. The most appropriate therapist response is to _____?

    1. refer the spouse to the director of rehabilitation
    2. refer the spouse to the client's primary physician
    3. refer the spouse to the client's primary nurse
    4. answer the spouse's question

37. A physical therapist prepares a presentation on proper body mechanics for a group of 100 autoworkers. Which of the following media would be most effective to maximize learning during the presentation?

    1. lecture, handouts
    2. lecture, charts, statistics
    3. lecture, handouts, demonstration
    4. lecture, statistics

38. A therapist prepares an inservice on repetitive use injuries for a group of administrative assistants. As part of the presentation, the therapist develops learning objectives. Which of the following objectives would be considered in the cognitive domain?

    1. List three potential consequences of an improperly designed work station.
    2. Correctly adjust the level of a computer keyboard.
    3. Devote five minutes in the morning and afternoon for stretching exercises.
    4. Demonstrate proper posture when sitting at a desk.

39. A physical therapist receives an order to devise a home program for a nine year old boy diagnosed with chondromalacia patella. As the therapist starts to explain the exercise instructions, it becomes obvious that the boy is not interested. Which of the following would be the most appropriate action to improve compliance with the home exercise program?

    1. Tell the boy he can leave because it is very difficult to help someone who does not want to be helped.
    2. Continue with the instructions hoping that the boy is a better listener than he appears to be.
    3. Lecture the boy on the importance of compliance with the home program.
    4. Ask a family member to come into the room while you explain the home program.

40. A therapist transports a brain injured client to the physical therapy gym. Each day after arriving in the gym, the client asks the therapist, "Where am I?" Recognizing the client has short term memory loss, the therapist's most appropriate response should be _____?

    1. You know where you are.
    2. You are in the same place you were yesterday at this time.
    3. You are in the physical therapy gym for your treatment session.
    4. You are in the hospital because of your injury.

D. Supporting Activities

Therapists should abide by established ethical and legal standards. They must demonstrate an awareness of the capabilities of supportive personnel and utilize their services in an appropriate fashion.

Ethical and Legal Standards

Ethical Decision Making
Standards of Practice
Confidentiality
Accountability
Malpractice
Tort

Scope of Practice
Code of Ethics
Informed Consent
Risk Management
Negligence

Delegation

Education
Training
Liability
Supervision
Physical Therapist Assistants
Other Support Personnel

Experience
Legality
Responsibility
Policies and Procedures
Physical Therapy Aides

Sample Questions

41. A physical therapist and a physical therapist assistant employed in an acute care hospital are responsible for providing weekend therapy coverage. After examining the client treatment list, the therapists attempt to develop an action plan. Which of the following activities would be the least appropriate for the physical therapist assistant?

    1. instruct a client in prosthetic donning and doffing
    2. assist a client with ambulation activities
    3. examine a client referred to physical therapy for instruction in a home exercise program
    4. perform goniometric measurements on a client two days status post anterior cruciate ligament reconstruction

42. A physical therapist fails to take into consideration a competent client's wishes when developing a treatment plan and the associated goals. Which of the following ethical principles has the therapist violated?

    1. autonomy
    2. beneficence
    3. nonmaleficence
    4. justice

43. A client rehabilitating from a fractured humerus has completed six weeks of physical therapy and is ready to be discharged with a home exercise program. The client is extremely pleased with his progress in therapy and gives the therapist a check for $50.00 as a token of his appreciation. The most appropriate therapist action is to _____?

    1. accept the money
    2. accept the money and donate it to charity
    3. accept the money and donate it to the department's general expense fund
    4. explain to the client that you are not permitted to accept money

44. A therapist awaiting the arrival of her next client observes another client ambulating independently in the parallel bars. The client appears to lack the necessary strength and coordination required to complete the activity independently. The therapist's most appropriate response would be to _____?

    1. inform the client's therapist of her observations
    2. assist the client back to a chair and contact the client's therapist
    3. ask the client if she is having difficulty or needs any assistance
    4. continue to observe the client, but do not interfere

45. Therapists often utilize information obtained in the clinical setting for a variety of educational purposes. Which of the following would represent an appropriate use of a medical record without client consent?

    1. informally discussing a client's medical record with another client
    2. permitting an unauthorized person access to a client's medical record
    3. utilization of the medical record as part of a quality assurance program
    4. research where anonymity is not preserved

E. System Specific Procedures

Procedures exist to treat selected systems of the body. The procedures are often a standard component of a physical therapy care plan. Therapists should be familiar with each of the selected procedures and understand their utilization as part of a treatment program.

Musculoskeletal

Joint Mobilization	Joint Manipulation
Soft Tissue Mobilization	Manual Traction
Connective Tissue Massage	Therapeutic Massage

Neuromuscular

Facilitation Techniques	Inhibition Techniques
Oral-Motor Stimulation	Vestibular Rehabilitation
Developmental Activities	Proprioceptive Neuromuscular Facilitation

Cardiopulmonary

Administer Oxygenation
Postural Drainage
Vibration
Suctioning
Respiratory Muscle Training

Assistive Cough Techniques

Breathing Exercises

Positioning
Percussion
Shaking
Incentive Spirometry
Intermittent Positive Pressure
Breathing
Techniques to Maximize
Ventilation
Bronchial Drainage

Integumentary

Debridement
Wet Dressings
Wound Cleansing

Dry Dressings
Topical Agents
Scar Management Techniques

Prosthetic Training

Residual Limb Care
Gait Training
Posture Training

Donning/Doffing
Balance Training
Exercise Programs

Sample Questions

46. A 32 year old female is admitted to the hospital after sustaining extensive burns to her trunk and right upper extremity. Which of the following burn classifications would most likely require the use of a graft?

    1. superficial burn
    2. superficial partial-thickness burn
    3. deep partial-thickness burn
    4. full-thickness burn

47. A therapist determines that a client is limited in right hip range of motion in a capsular pattern. If the therapist elects to focus on increasing hip flexion, which mobilization techniques would be indicated?

    1. anterior glide
    2. posterior glide
    3. lateral glide
    4. medial glide

↑ hip flex + IR

Convex on concave

48. An order for chest physical therapy is received for an 82 year old female. The client recently underwent surgery for a hip fracture and has been taking Coumadin postoperatively. She has a history of multiple compression fractures of the thoracic vertebrae. The greatest amount of caution should be taken in the administration of _____?

   1. diaphragmatic breathing exercises
   2. postural drainage
   3. therapeutic percussion
   4. pursed lip breathing

49. A client who sustained a deep laceration in the antecubital fossa is treated in physical therapy. The client's wound has been healing poorly secondary to motion occurring at the elbow joint. Which type of dressing would be the most appropriate to facilitate wound healing?

   1. wet
   2. dry
   3. occlusive
   4. rigid

50. A therapist utilizes joint mobilization techniques for pain control and muscle relaxation at the shoulder. If the therapist begins by mobilizing the glenohumeral joint in the resting position, the limb should be positioned in _____?

   1. 55 degrees of abduction, 30 degrees of horizontal adduction
   2. 30 degrees of abduction, 10 degrees of horizontal adduction
   3. 25 degrees of abduction, 5 degrees of horizontal abduction
   4. 10 degrees of adduction, 5 degrees of horizontal abduction

General Principles

The health care delivery system and issues associated with research activities are not identified in one specific subtopic. Instead, these topics are infused throughout each of the three content areas. It is important for therapists to possess a thorough understanding of both of these topics. Sample questions based on the health care delivery system and research activities are presented throughout the text.

Health Care Delivery System

Management Principles	Policies and Procedures
Quality Assurance	Utilization Review
Dispute Resolution	Time Management
Budgeting	Marketing
Scheduling	Performance Evaluation
Staff Resources	Program Development
Continuing Education	Strategic Plan
HMO	Preferred Provider Network
Worker's Compensation	Medicaid
Medicare	Self Insured
Fee for Service	Capitation

Evaluate/Participate in Research Activities

Types of Research

Review of Literature

Institutional Review Board

Data Collection

Statistical Significance

Dissemination

Research Design

Research Proposal

Informed Consent

Statistical Analysis

Clinical Relevance

[1] Adapted from PT Test Content Outline, Federation of State Boards of Physical Therapy, 1997

Answer Key

1. Answer: 4   Resource: Goodman (25)

   Leading questions may serve to bias a client and often can generate erroneous information. Questions that are very specific have a tendency to be leading.

2. Answer: 1   Resource: Booher (525)

   The injury mechanism associated with an acromioclavicular injury is a direct blow to the tip of the shoulder which serves to displace the acromion inferior to the clavicle.

3. Answer: 4   Resource: Magee (41)

   Although x-rays can be used to assess skeletal maturity, the primary purpose would be to rule out a fracture.

4. Answer: 1   Resource: Guide for Professional Conduct

   The therapist's hypothesis necessitates contact with the referring physician, however does not indicate the need to discontinue physical therapy services.

5. Answer: 1   Resource: Goodman (431)

   Headaches occur in 30% - 50% of clients with brain tumors. Visual changes can be caused by space occupying tumors.

6. Answer: 1   Resource: Hoppenfeld (216)

   The sinus tarsi area is located immediately anterior to the lateral malleolus. The soft tissue depression consists of a tunnel between the calcaneus and talus.

7. Answer: 2   Resource: Hertling (85)

   Sensory testing for light touch is performed by applying the piece of cotton to selected dermatomes and asking the client when the sensation is perceived.

8. Answer: 4   Resource: Shumway-Cook (67)

Abnormalities of the vestibular system result in dizziness and impaired balance. The vestibular system itself is stimulated by the position of the head in space and changes in the direction of movement of the head.

9. Answer: 4   Resource: Hoppenfeld (254)

The Achilles reflex is from the S1 level. Sensation on the posterior calf is from the S1-S2 level while the bowel is associated with the sacral segments of the spinal cord S2-S4.

10. Answer: 3   Resource: Magee (479)

Measuring from the medial knee joint line to the medial malleolus allows for an independent assessment of tibial length and also avoids any potential asymmetries due to leg girth.

11. Answer: 2   Resource: Hertling (535)

The therapist should clear the client's vertebral artery for his/her available range of motion. As the client gains additional range of motion the test can be readministered. It is possible to observe findings such as nystagmus and slurring of speech prior to achieving full rotation, extension and lateral flexion.

12. Answer: 3   Resource: Brannon (226)

ST segment depression of less than 1 mm may occur in a healthy individual during exercise.

13. Answer: 2   Resource: Magee (483)

This scenario describes Ely's test which if positive is indicative of tightness of the two joint hip flexor.

14. Answer: 3   Resource: Pierson (47)

The radial artery offers a convenient site to assess pulse while a 30 second interval provides the opportunity to secure an accurate measurement without allowing for a full recovery from exercise.

15. Answer: 1   Resource: Magee (572)

Patellar L3-L4, lateral hamstrings S1-S2, posterior tibial L4-L5, Achilles S1-S2.

16. Answer: 2   Resource: Ellis (31)

Pressure on the patella is likely due to the residual limb pistoning in the socket. A one ply sock may stop the pistoning and allow the weight bearing forces to be absorbed by the patellar tendon.

17. Answer: 3   Resource: Clark (343)

Since the client has a sensory alteration and ambulating a distance of only sixty feet created irritation, it is advisable to avoid utilizing the orthosis until modifications are made.

18. Answer: 4   Resource: Roy (118)

The information does not include data from the uninvolved lower extremity. Other necessary information might include ability to complete a functional progression, ROM, edema, etc.

19. Answer: 4   Resource: Paz (376)

The client's signs and symptoms are consistent with the presence of a deep venous thrombosis. Referral for additional examination is necessary.

20. Answer: 4   Resource: Kisner (571)

The packages may be too heavy or the conveyor belt may be too high. In both cases the task is too difficult.

21. Answer: 3   Resource: Post-Stroke Rehabilitation (74)

The client needs additional therapy services and appears to fit the definition of homebound. Based on her postoperative status and the surgical procedure more intensive therapy services does not seem warranted.

22. Answer: 4   Resource: Brannon (3)

Activities in a phase I cardiac rehabilitation program typically progress to 3 METs.

23. Answer: 2   Resource: Kettenbach (96)

The client appears to be making progress through the established short term goals and by developing additional, perhaps more directed short term goals it may facilitate achievement of the long term goal. Not enough information is given to assume the long term goal is unrealistic particularly since the client is making progress.

24. Answer: 4   Resource: Standards of Practice

The client has achieved all established short and long term goals and has returned to his previous lifestyle. There is no longer a need for physical therapy services.

25. Answer: 2   Resource: Scott - Health Care Malpractice (133)

Although each of the options are viable answers, the therapist's primary responsibility is direct client care. Failure to provide physical therapy services for this period of time in an acute care environment could pose a serious problem.

26. Answer: 3   Resource: Rothstein (24)

For each inch of vertical rise a properly constructed ramp will have 12 inches of length.

27. Answer: 4   Resource: Guide to Physical Therapist
                                                                                    Practice

The physician is responsible for determining when the sling can be discontinued.

28. Answer: 3   Resource: Thomas (1992)

The Trendelenburg position is an inclined position in which the body and legs are elevated in relation to the head. This position is not recommended with clients with a known or suspected head injury.

29. Answer: 4   Resource: Kisner (634)

Clients with chronic arterial insufficiency typically have diminished blood flow and resultant ischemia. Dependent positioning such as having the legs elevated will only serve to exacerbate the client's symptoms.

30. Answer: 2   Resource: Robinson (75)

Electrical equipment should be inspected at a minimum on an annual basis.

31. Answer: 4   Resource: Thomas (951)

The most immediate response should be to eliminate the causative factor which is the positional change. Therefore it is necessary to lower the tilt table.

32. Answer: 4   Resource: Michlovitz (142)

A warm water bath is the most appropriate superficial heating agent to incorporate into the home program since it is readily available and easily applied to the lower leg and foot.

33. Answer: 1   Resource: De Domenico (9)

Effleurage is defined as passing the hands over a large body area through gentle or deep stroking. Effleurage is often used as an initial, transitional, and/or final massage technique.

34. Answer: 2   Resource: Kisner (89)

The first set consists of ten repetitions at 50% of the 10 repetition maximum.
10RM = 80 pounds   50% of 80 pounds = 40 pounds

35. Answer: 3   Resource: Minor (314)

Pushing up on the chair with both hands provides the most stable base to achieve a standing position. It is important not to reach for the walker while standing since it may have a tendency to move the client's center of gravity outside his/her base of support.

36. Answer: 4   Resource: Guide for Professional Conduct

The question asked by the spouse falls within the therapist's scope of practice and should therefore be answered directly.

37. Answer: 3   Resource: Haggard (83)

Lecture, handouts and demonstration provide not only verbal and written information, but provide the target audience with the opportunity to observe an actual demonstration. This multitiered approach accomodates a variety of learning styles.

38. Answer: 1   Resource: Arends (47)

Domains of learning include Cognitive, Affective and Psychomotor. Bloom's Taxonomy of Educational Objectives identifies six levels of the cognitive domain: knowledge, comprehension, application, analysis, synthesis and evaluation.

39. Answer: 4   Resource: Davis (208)

Due to the client's age it would be appropriate to ask a family member to come into the room. To reprimand the boy in any form may only serve to diminish compliance.

40. Answer: 3   Resource: O'Sullivan (502)

A client's question should be answered in a direct and forthcoming manner whenever possible. Frequent repetition is a component of any treatment plan for clients with short term memory loss.

41. Answer: 3   Resource: Guide to Physical Therapist
                                                               Practice

Physical therapist assistants perform procedures and related tasks that have been selected and delegated by the supervising physical therapist. It is not appropriate to delegate an examination.

42. Answer: 1   Resource: Davis (61)

Autonomy is defined as independent functioning. As an ethical term it indicates freedom to decide or freedom to act.

43. Answer: 4   Resource: Guide to Professional Conduct

The code of ethics states that "physical therapists seek reimbursement for their services that is deserved and reasonable." Accepting a check from a client, regardless of its use is unacceptable.

44. Answer: 2   Resource: Guide for Professional Conduct

The therapist has made a judgment that the client "lacks the necessary strength and coordination required to complete the activity independently." The only method to resolve the situation and be sure the client is unharmed is to become directly involved.

45. Answer: 3   Resource: Walter (244)

Quality assurance programs are an internal process aimed at improving client care, therefore client consent is not necessary.

46. Answer: 4   Resource: Rothstein (1117)

Full thickness burns are characterized by complete destruction of the epidermis and dermis with or without damage to the subcutaneous fat layer. Since new tissue is only generated from the periphery of the burn site, grafts are necessary.

47. Answer: 2   Resource: Kisner (221)

A posterior glide of the femur on the acetabulum is indicated to increase flexion and internal rotation.

48. Answer: 3   Resource: Irwin (345)

Percussion is a technique that can be used to mobilize retained secretions. The technique involves direct contact over a given segment of the lung and should therefore be used with caution based on the client's past medical history.

49. Answer: 4   Resource: Trofino (43)

A rigid dressing will serve to immobilize the injured area and offer protection from outside contaminants.

50. Answer: 1   Resource: Magee (175)

The glenohumeral joint is a ball and socket **joint** that has three axes and three degrees of freedom. The close packed position is full abduction and lateral rotation.

Unit Seven
Final Preparation

As the date of the Physical Therapist Examination steadily approaches, candidates usually experience an increase in their anxiety level. Candidates often voice concerns such as: "How am I going to remember everything?" "What if I studied the wrong material?" or "Did I study enough?" Unfortunately, the answer to these seemingly simple questions can be very complicated.

The good news is that candidates who have taken the time to develop a comprehensive study plan and periodically have assessed their progress towards meeting established goals, tend to perform well on the examination. The performance of candidates who have either neglected to study or have approached their studying in a random or inefficient manner can be much more difficult to predict.

Regardless of which description best describes your preparation, when the examination is less than 48 hours away, it is simply too late to make any significant changes in your study plan. Instead, candidates need to focus on other variables they can control. This unit will offer specific suggestions for candidates to incorporate into their final preparation.

Examination Strategy

Just as you developed an individualized study plan according to your needs as a learner, you now need to consider how you can take the examination with the same considerations in mind.

If you determined you were an Active/Active or Active/Passive learner for input and processing, you may find this four hour, physically passive testing environment particularly trying and consequently, anxiety producing. You may find yourself being distracted by every noise, vibration, and movement in the room, and may notice that your ability to concentrate has been compromised. Although it is impossible to have the same type of control over the examination site as you did over your study sessions, it is possible to make a few alterations which can be beneficial:

1. Attempt to secure a corner location. Corner locations tend to limit peripheral vision distracters.
2. Consider wearing earplugs to block out some of the unnecessary background noise.
3. Chewing gum or sucking on hard candy may be soothing.
4. Prior to beginning the examination write down question numbers 25, 50, 75, 100, 125, 150, 175 and 200 on a piece of paper and place it in a visible location. As you progress through the examination, perform a brief relaxation exercise at each of the scheduled intervals. A sample relaxation exercise is outlined in the Appendix.

If you determined you were a Passive/Active or Passive/Passive learner you may not be as challenged by the physically passive nature of the four hour testing environment, but the intensity of the mental activity may produce anxiety in the form of tense muscles and a gradual lengthening of the time needed to answer each question. Here are some recommendations you may consider:

1. Choose a location in front of the room to avoid being disturbed by the movements of other candidates.
2. If you concentrate better in a quiet setting, you may want to consider wearing earplugs.
3. Prior to beginning the examination write down question number 50, 100, 150, and 200 on a piece of paper and place it in a visible location. As you progress through the examination, perform the relaxation exercise at each of the sheduled intervals. A sample relaxation exercise is outlined in the Appendix.

The suggested recommendations for each learning style should be incorporated into a candidate's study plan. Candidates can attempt to incorporate the recommendations as they take the 200 question sample examination located in Unit Eight. By utilizing this information prior to the actual examination, candidates can evaluate the utility of each suggestion and construct an individualized examination strategy.

Miscellaneous Items

Examination Site

If candidates are not familiar with the exact location of the examination site, it is often prudent to travel to the site before the actual examination date. This trip can serve two important purposes. The first is that candidates will have an accurate idea of the time necessary to travel to the site, and therefore will be able to plan accordingly the day of the examination. The second purpose is that the pre-examination visit should eliminate the possibility of getting lost and subsequently being late for the examination.

Studying

Last minute studying is strongly discouraged. Candidates should avoid studying the entire day before the examination. A 24 hour period without studying is often necessary to put the mind at ease and limit needless worry about the examination. Candidates who have prepared adequately will feel comfortable with their preparation and will go into the examination with a high level of confidence. Last minute studying only will serve to undermine this confidence.

Testing Supplies

Take time the day prior to the examination to gather the necessary supplies. Although the exact supply list may vary depending on individual state requirements, it is recommended that candidates bring to the examination the following supplies: two writing utensils; two forms of identification including one which is a photo, such as a driver's license; and a confirmation registration card. It is important to emphasize, however, that individual state requirements can differ and candidates should take special care to meet each requirement.

Dress

Plan to dress comfortably for the examination. Select an outfit the night before that can be altered depending on conditions at the examination site. Generally a blouse or shirt with a sweater can accommodate to a variety of conditions. Pants are generally the preferred choice over shorts. Light pants tend to be comfortable in warm weather and also keep the chill off in air conditioning or colder conditions.

Although your clothing will not determine your examination score, it is important to be comfortable. Excessive heat or cold can serve as distracters during the examination.

Entertainment

The night before the examination, engage in an activity that you particularly enjoy, whether it's going to your favorite restaurant, a theater performance, or spending a quiet evening at home with your significant other. By taking part in a planned activity, you will avoid focusing on the impending examination and harness any growing anxiety.

Bedtime

Make a special effort to be in bed at or before your usual time. Your mind will need to be rested and at optimal functioning level the day of the examination. Lack of sleep or other deterrents, such as alcohol or drugs will serve to limit your performance. Use an alarm clock to make sure you are up in plenty of time on the big day.

The Big Day

As the blare of the alarm clock breaks the morning calm, your day officially begins. Since you already have performed the majority of the tasks associated with the licensing examination, there should be little extra to do except your routine daily activities.

Special attention should be given to eating well balanced meals. Considering there will be some travel associated with getting to the examination site, and the allotted examination time is four hours, it may be quite awhile until you have the opportunity to eat again.

Travel

Be sure to leave extra time when traveling to the Sylvan Technology Center. Leaving additional time will allow a candidate to enter the examination site calm and collected. Arriving late or just as the examination is scheduled to begin will cause needless stress and may have a negative impact on a candidate's performance.

Show Time

Always take the available time to review the tutorial prior to beginning the examination. The fifteen minutes allotted to the tutorial does not count toward the four hour time period given to take the actual examination. Be sure that you have a thorough understanding of the information conveyed in the tutorial prior to beginning the examination. If anything remains unclear, seek additional guidance from an authorized Sylvan agent. The tutorial not only reminds you of several important features of computer based testing, but also can serve as a way to limit growing test anxiety.

When taking the actual examination, read all questions carefully and consider each option with an open mind. Finish the examination only when you either have used all of the allotted time or have finished reviewing your work. When leaving the examination take solace knowing that you did the best job possible. Take pride in the fact your preparation was both timely and effective. Resist the temptation to scrutinize and second guess yourself; it will only result in wasted energy and cannot possibly change your examination results. Typically, candidates will be notified of their results in two to four weeks by their state licensing agency.

Conclusion

We have presented a number of different strategies that, when used appropriately, can assist candidates to maximize their performance on the Physical Therapist Examination. Candidates should avoid focusing on any of the specific strategies in isolation, and instead incorporate them into a comprehensive study plan.

Candidates should attempt to develop methods to expand their study plan beyond the scope of the material we have presented. One example of this would be by utilizing the content outline. Throughout the text we have offered our interpretation of each subcategory of the content outline. Candidates should attempt to generate their own interpretation of each subcategory and speculate on what type of material might be contained within its boundaries. By doing this, candidates will acquire a deeper and more comprehensive understanding of the material on the Physical Therapist Examination.

By utilizing the information contained in our text and developing specific individual strategies, you already have taken a large step towards being successful on the Physical Therapist Examination.

Unit Eight
Sample Examination

As we have indicated numerous times throughout this text, candidates can obtain a great deal of valuable information by taking sample examinations. Candidates who are exposed to sample examinations have several distinct opportunities that otherwise may not be available.

1. Candidates have the opportunity to refine their test taking skills with sample questions that are similar in design and format to actual examination questions.

2. Candidates have the opportunity to assess their current level of preparation prior to the actual examination.

In this unit, candidates will have the opportunity to take a 200 question sample examination. In order to assess a candidate's performance on the sample examination, a number of indicators must be examined. Perhaps the most obvious indicator is the number of questions a candidate answers correctly. Since the Physical Therapist Examination consists of 200 questions, the maximum number of questions a candidate can answer correctly is 200. The established criterion-referenced score for the 200 question sample examination is 155.

Unfortunately, it is not possible to identify a single number of questions that must be answered correctly in order to be successful on the actual Physical Therapist Examination. This number fluctuates based on the level of difficulty of each given examination. Candidates should use the number of questions answered correctly on the sample examination only as a general indicator of their current level of preparation.

There are a number of less obvious indicators that can offer candidates feedback as they prepare for the Physical Therapist Examination. These indicators often are best examined by answering several selected questions.

- Were you able to maintain the same level of concentration throughout the entire examination?

- Did you have adequate time to complete the examination?

- Did you effectively incorporate test taking strategies?

- Did you misinterpret or fail to identify what selected questions were asking?

- Did the questions that were answered incorrectly exhibit any similar characteristics?

- Did you make any careless mistakes?

Exercise

Each candidate will have a maximum of four hours to complete the 200 question examination. Candidates should attempt to take the examination in a single designated four hour period. By completing the examination in this fashion, candidates can make the sample examination more realistic, and therefore will be able to gather more accurate information on their performance.

Attempt to identify the best answer to each question and mark the answer in the appropriate space on the accompanying answer sheets. After completing the examination, utilize the answer key located at the conclusion of the exercise to determine the number of questions answered correctly.

The criterion-referenced passing score for the sample examination is 155. Therefore a score of 155 or more would be a passing score and a score of less than 155 would be a failing score.

SAMPLE PHYSICAL THERAPIST EXAMINATION

1. A therapist instructs a client rehabilitating from a tibial plateau fracture to ascend a curb using axillary crutches. The client is partial weightbearing and uses a three point gait pattern when ambulating. When ascending a curb the therapist should instruct the client to lead with the _____?

   1. uninvolved lower extremity
   2. involved lower extremity
   3. axillary crutches
   4. right axillary crutch and right lower extremity

2. A therapist attempts to transfer a moderately obese client from a wheelchair to a bed. The therapist is concerned about the size of the client, but is unable to secure another staff member to assist with the transfer. Which type of transfer would allow the therapist to move the client with the greatest ease?

   1. dependent standing pivot
   2. hydraulic lift
   3. sliding board
   4. assisted standing pivot

3. A therapist conducts a goniometric assessment of a client's upper extremities. Which of the following values is most indicative of normal passive glenohumeral abduction?

   1. 80 degrees
   2. 120 degrees
   3. 155 degrees
   4. 180 degrees

   60° occuring at Scapulothoracic Jt

4. A therapist designs a therapeutic exercise program for a client with sway-back. The most appropriate exercise is _____?

   lordosis

   1. lower abdominal strengthening
   2. hip flexor strengthening
   3. anterior pelvic tilts
   4. lower back strengthening

5. A therapist monitors a client's respiration rate during exercise. Which of the following would be considered a normal response?

   1. the respiration rate declines during exercise before the intensity of exercise declines
   2. the respiration rate does not increase during exercise
   3. the rhythm of the respiration pattern becomes irregular during exercise
   4. the respiration rate decreases as the intensity of the exercise plateaus

6. A therapist reviews the results of a pulmonary function test. Assuming normal values, which of the following measurements would you expect to be the greatest?

    1. vital capacity
    2. tidal volume
    3. residual volume
    4. inspiratory reserve volume

7. A client involved in a motor vehicle accident sustains an injury to the posterior cord of the brachial plexus. Which muscle would not be affected by the injury?

    1. infraspinatus
    2. subscapularis
    3. latissimus dorsi
    4. teres major

8. While treating a client bedside, a therapist notices that an improperly positioned bedrail has partially occluded the tubing of an IV line. The therapist's most immediate response should be to _____?

    1. contact nursing
    2. contact the referring physician
    3. reposition the bedrail
    4. document the incident

9. A therapist designs a training program for a client without cardiovascular pathology. The therapist calculates the client's age predicted maximal heart rate as 175 beats per minute. Which of the following would be an acceptable target heart rate for the client during cardiovascular exercise?

    1. 93 beats per minute
    2. 122 beats per minute
    3. 169 beats per minute
    4. 195 beats per minute

10. While preparing a sterile field for wound debridement, a therapist accidentally places a nonsterile object on the sterile base. The most appropriate action is to _____?

    1. remove the nonsterile object from the sterile base and continue with treatment
    2. continue with treatment; however, be sure no other supplies come in contact with the nonsterile object
    3. remove all of the items to be used from the sterile base and replace them with similar items that are sterile
    4. discard the entire sterile field and establish a new sterile field

114

11. A client rehabilitating from a fractured right humerus is examined in physical therapy. The therapist determines goniometrically that the client can actively flex his right shoulder to 173 degrees. Which of the following entries would be the most appropriate to illustrate the therapist's findings?

    1. right shoulder flexion range of motion 0 - 173 degrees
    2. right shoulder range of motion is within normal limits
    3. right shoulder flexion active range of motion to 173 degrees
    4. right shoulder active range of motion to 173 degrees

12. A therapist works with a client placed in isolation. The therapist is required to wear a mask while treating the client, but is not required to wear gloves or a gown. This type of isolation could be termed _____?

    1. strict isolation
    2. contact isolation
    3. respiratory isolation
    4. blood/body fluid precautions

13. A 13 year old female diagnosed with cerebral palsy is referred to physical therapy. The client exhibits slow, involuntary, continuous writhing movements of the upper and lower extremities. This type of motor disturbance best describes _____?

    1. spasticity
    2. ataxia
    3. hypotonia
    4. athetosis

14. A client, who is status post stroke and demonstrates Wernicke's aphasia, is learning how to perform a sit to stand transfer. To enhance the client's ability to learn the transfer, the physical therapist should avoid _____ when instructing the client?

    1. using a mirror for visual feedback
    2. providing detailed instructions
    3. using repetition
    4. demonstrating

15. A physician refers a client rehabilitating from a fractured femur to physical therapy for gait training. Which of the following would not be the responsibility of the physical therapist?

    1. assessing balance
    2. determining weightbearing status
    3. selecting an assistive device
    4. assessing endurance

16. The Occupational Safety and Health Administration establishes regulations for health care facilities, which are designed to protect their employees. Which of the following regulations is not accurate?

    1. Provide proper containers for the disposal of waste and sharp items.
    2. Educate employees on the methods of transmission and the prevention of hepatitis B and HIV.
    3. Require all employees to receive the hepatitis B vaccine.
    4. Provide education and follow up care to employees who are exposed to communicable diseases.

17. A client status post total hip replacement is referred to physical therapy for gait training. The client has not been weightbearing on the involved lower extremity since surgery and appears to be somewhat anxious. The most appropriate setting to begin ambulation activities is _____?

    1. in the parallel bars
    2. in the parallel bars with a rolling walker
    3. in the physical therapy gym with a straight cane
    4. in the physical therapy gym with a walker

18. A client involved in a motor vehicle accident sustains a Colles' fracture and an intertrochanteric hip fracture. The client has been cleared for touch-down weight bearing by her physician. Which assistive device would be the most appropriate for the client?

    1. straight cane
    2. axillary crutches
    3. rolling walker
    4. walker with a platform attachment

19. A therapist instructs a 55 year old trauma victim with bilateral lower extremity paralysis to transfer from a wheelchair to a mat table. The client has normal upper extremity strength and has no other known medical problems. The most appropriate transfer technique is a _____?

    1. dependent standing pivot
    2. sliding board transfer
    3. two person carry
    4. hydraulic lift

20. A therapist elects to utilize joint mobilization to increase the extensibility of the ulnohumeral joint. Which position of the ulnohumeral joint would be inappropriate for joint mobilization?

    1. 15 degrees extension, 15 degrees pronation
    2. 70 degrees flexion, 10 degrees supination
    3. 30 degrees flexion, 25 degrees supination
    4. full extension and supination — Close packed

21. A therapist instructs a client to make a fist. The client can make a fist, but is unable to flex the distal phalanx of the ring finger. This clinical finding can best be explained by _____?

    1. a ruptured flexor carpi radialis tendon
    2. a ruptured flexor digitorum superficialis tendon
    3. a ruptured flexor digitorum profundus tendon
    4. a ruptured extensor digitorum communis tendon

22. A client with a confirmed posterior cruciate ligament tear is able to return to full dynamic activities following rehabilitation. Which of the following does not serve as a secondary restraint to the posterior cruciate ligament?

    1. iliotibial band
    2. popliteus
    3. lateral collateral ligament
    4. medial collateral ligament

23. A nine month old infant with cerebral palsy is unable to roll from prone to supine. This developmental activity typically occurs by _____?

    1. 3 months
    2. 5 months
    3. 7 months
    4. 9 months

24. A physical therapist working in a school system develops long term goals as part of an Individualized Educational Plan for a child with Down's Syndrome. The most appropriate time frame for these goals is _____?

    1. one month
    2. four months
    3. six months
    4. one year

25. A therapist administers ultrasound over a client's anterior thigh. After one minute of treatment, the client reports feeling a slight burning sensation under the sound head. The therapist's most appropriate action is to _____?

    1. explain to the client that what she feels is not out of the ordinary when using ultrasound
    2. temporarily discontinue treatment and examine the amount of coupling
    3. discontinue treatment and contact the referring physician
    4. continue with treatment utilizing the current parameters

117

26. A client is positioned on a treatment table in prone with two pillows under her hips. This position most likely would be used to perform postural drainage techniques to the _____?

   1. anterior basal segment of the lower lobes
   2. lateral basal segment of the lower lobes
   3. right middle lobe
   4. superior segment of the lower lobes

27. A client eight weeks post myocardial infarction is involved in a phase II cardiac rehabilitation program at a local hospital. What event usually signifies the completion of a phase II program?

   1. echocardiogram
   2. initiation of a high level aerobic exercise program
   3. low level treadmill test
   4. maximal treadmill test

28. A client being treated in an outpatient orthopedic clinic begins to demonstrate signs and symptoms of stroke, including sudden weakness of the arm and leg, unexplained dizziness, and loss of vision. Recognizing the symptoms of a stroke the therapist begins to administer first aid. Which of the following would not be considered appropriate first aid management?

   1. monitor the airway, breathing, and circulation
   2. remove mucus from the mouth with a piece of cloth wrapped around a finger
   3. position the client in supine and slightly elevate the legs
   4. immediately contact medical assistance

29. Pharmacological agents eventually must be eliminated from the body to prevent an excessive accumulation of a specific drug. Where is the major site for drug excretion?

   1. gastrointestinal tract *+ lungs are 2° sites*
   2. kidneys
   3. liver
   4. saliva

30. A therapist designs an exercise program for a pregnant woman. Which of the following exercises would be inappropriate?

   1. pelvic floor isometrics
   2. squatting
   3. standing push-ups
   4. bilateral straight leg raising

31. A therapist treats a client with generalized upper and lower extremity weakness
following a prolonged hospitalization. As part of the client's treatment program,
the therapist designs an aquatic program emphasizing upper and lower extremity
range of motion. Which physical property of water allows the client to move with
greater ease?

1. buoyancy
2. specific gravity
3. specific heat
4. thermal conductivity

32. A therapist examines a grossly obese client referred to physical therapy with a hip
flexor strain. Which modality would have the greatest ability to elevate the
temperature of fatty tissue to potentially dangerous levels?

1. diathermy
2. hot packs
3. paraffin
4. pulsed ultrasound

33. A 66 year old female is referred to physical therapy with rheumatoid arthritis.
During the initial examination the therapist notes increased flexion at the proximal
interphalangeal joints and hyperextension at the metacarpophalangeal and distal
interphalangeal joints. This deformity commonly is known as _____?

1. boutonniere deformity
2. mallet finger
3. swan neck deformity
4. ulnar drift

34. A therapist discusses the importance of proper nutrition with a client diagnosed with
congestive heart failure. Which of the following substances would be most
restricted in this client's diet?

1. cholesterol
2. potassium
3. sodium
4. triglycerides

35. A physician reduces a comminuted tibia fracture using an external fixation device.
Which stage of bone healing is associated with the termination of external fixation?

1. hematoma formation
2. cellular proliferation
3. callus formation
4. clinical union

36. A 62 year old male diagnosed with ankylosing spondylitis is referred to physical therapy. The client's referral is for instruction in a home exercise program. Which of the following exercises would you expect to be the most appropriate for this client?

    1. partial sit ups
    2. posterior pelvic tilts
    3. spinal extension
    4. straight leg raises

37. A client diagnosed with piriformis syndrome is referred to physical therapy for one visit for instruction in a home exercise program. After examining the client, the therapist feels the client's rehabilitation potential is excellent, but is concerned that one visit will not be sufficient to meet the client's needs. The most appropriate action is to _____?

    1. schedule the client for treatment sessions, as warranted, based on the results of the initial examination
    2. explain to the client that recent health care reforms have drastically reduced the frequency of physical therapy visits covered by third party payers
    3. explain to the client that she can continue with physical therapy beyond the initial session, but will be liable for all expenses not covered by her insurance
    4. contact the referring physician and request approval for additional physical therapy visits

38. A male client with limited shoulder range of motion explains that he has difficulty wiping himself after going to the bathroom. How much shoulder range of motion is required to successfully complete toileting activities?

    1. 50 degrees horizontal abduction, 30 degrees abduction, 45 degrees medial rotation
    2. 30 degrees horizontal abduction, 45 degrees adduction, 65 degrees medial rotation
    3. 80 degrees horizontal abduction, 40 degrees abduction, 90 degrees medial rotation
    4. 90 degrees horizontal adduction, 75 degrees abduction, 60 degrees medial rotation

39. A therapist completes lower extremity range of motion activities with a spinal cord injured client. While ranging the client, the therapist notices that the client's urine is extremely dark and has a distinctive foul smelling odor. Which of the following is the most appropriate action?

    1. verbally report the observation to the client's physician
    2. verbally report the observation to the client's nurse
    3. document and verbally report the observation to the client's nurse
    4. document and verbally report the observation to the director of rehabilitation

40. An eight year old female with a 25 degree scoliotic curve is fitted for a Milwaukee brace. The brace will likely be worn until _____?

   1. the scoliotic curve does not increase within a one year period
   2. the client resumes all recreational and athletic activities
   3. the client is pain free for six months
   4. spinal growth ceases

41. Clients with abnormal conduction patterns often can be treated successfully using antiarrhythmic medication. Which of the following side effects of antiarrythmics would not require immediate medical attention?

   1. dizziness
   2. insomnia
   3. shortness of breath
   4. coughing up blood

42. A therapist uses a S.O.A.P. note format for all of his daily documentation. Which of the following would not be found in the assessment section of a S.O.A.P. note?

   1. short and long term goals
   2. discussion of a client's progress in therapy
   3. client's equipment needs and equipment ordered Plan
   4. client's rehabilitation potential

43. A rehabilitation manager designs a system to monitor the productivity of staff therapists. Which piece of data would be the least beneficial to accomplish the manager's objective?

   1. number of generated timed treatment units
   2. results of client satisfaction survey data
   3. total hours of direct client treatment time
   4. number of regular payroll hours

44. A 52 year old, self referred male is examined in physical therapy. The client states that over the last three months he has experienced increasing neck stiffness and pain at night. He also communicates that within the past week he has had several episodes of dizziness. The client has a family history of cancer and has smoked two packs of cigarettes a day for the last twenty years. The client denies any other significant past medical history and lists the date of his last medical examination as 10 years ago. The therapist's most appropriate action is to _____?

   1. treat the client conservatively and document any changes in the client's status
   2. inform the client that he is not a candidate for physical therapy
   3. refer the client to an oncologist
   4. refer the client to his primary care physician

45. Therapists use a wide variety of measurement methods in their daily documentation. These measurements usually are categorized as subjective or objective methods. Which of the following measurement methods would not be considered objective?

    1. duration of attention
    2. goniometric measurements
    3. rating on a perceived exertion scale
    4. time required to perform a selected activity

46. Therapists often begin the interview process with a new client by using open-ended questions. Which of the following questions would not be considered open-ended?

    1. What makes your pain better?
    2. Is your back more painful at night?
    3. How does exercise affect your back?
    4. Describe your activities in a typical day.

47. A client is referred to physical therapy following surgery to repair a torn rotator cuff. The physician referral does not include postoperative guidelines and also does not classify the extent or size of the tear. The therapist's most appropriate action is to _____?

    1. consult various medical resources that discuss physical therapy management of rotator cuff repairs
    2. consult various protocols of other surgeons in the area
    3. contact the referring physician and discuss the client's care
    4. discuss the client's care with other staff members who are more experienced in treating rotator cuff repairs

48. A client with chronic shoulder instability is scheduled to have an open Bankart procedure. As part of the surgery, the subscapularis is removed and then reattached to the anterior capsule. In order to protect the subscapularis postoperatively, which of the following shoulder motions initially should be most limited?

    1. flexion
    2. abduction
    3. internal rotation
    4. external rotation

49. A client paralyzed from the waist down discusses accessibility issues with an employer in preparation for her return to work. The client is concerned about her ability to navigate a wheelchair in certain areas of the building. What is the minimum space required to turn 180 degrees in a standard wheelchair?

    1. 32 inches
    2. 48 inches
    3. 60 inches
    4. 72 inches

50. A client is scheduled to undergo a transtibial amputation secondary to poor healing of an ulcer on his left foot. In addition, the client is two months status post right knee replacement due to osteoarthritis. Given the client's past and current medical history, the physical therapist can expect which of the following tasks to be the most difficult for the client following his amputation?

    1. rolling from supine to sidelying
    2. moving from sitting to supine
    3. moving from sitting to standing
    4. ambulating in the parallel bars

51. A therapist wears sterile protective clothing while treating a client. Which area of the protective clothing would not be considered sterile even before coming in contact with a nonsterile object?

    1. gloves
    2. sleeves of the gown
    3. front of the gown above waist level
    4. front of the gown below waist level

52. A therapist conducts goniometric measurements on a client in supine. When measuring elbow flexion the therapist's stabilizing force should be directed at the _____?

    1. radioulnar joint
    2. olecranon
    3. distal humerus 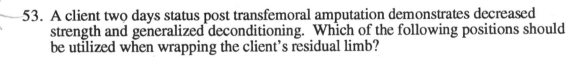 to prevent shld flex
    4. proximal humerus

53. A client two days status post transfemoral amputation demonstrates decreased strength and generalized deconditioning. Which of the following positions should be utilized when wrapping the client's residual limb?

    1. sidelying
    2. standing
    3. supine
    4. prone

54. A client who underwent a transtibial amputation one week ago complains of phantom sensation. Which of the following treatment options would be inappropriate?

    1. tell the client to leave the residual limb exposed to the air at all times
    2. discuss the option of a temporary prosthesis with the client's physician
    3. begin residual limb wrapping
    4. teach the client to tap and massage the residual limb

55. A therapist transports a client with multiple sclerosis to the gym for her treatment session. The client is wheelchair dependent and uses a urinary catheter. When transporting the client, the most appropriate location to secure the collection bag is _____?

   1. in the client's lap
   2. on the lower abdomen
   3. on the wheelchair armrest
   4. on the wheelchair legrest

56. A physical therapist examines a client with multiple sclerosis. The client has poor to fair strength in her legs, good arm strength, and moderate truncal ataxia. The safest means for the client to ambulate in her home would be _____?

   1. with a single point cane
   2. with a walker
   3. while holding onto furniture or walls
   4. with axillary crutches

57. A physical therapist attempts to examine the extent of ataxia in a client's upper extremities. The preferred method to examine and document ataxia is _____?

   1. manual muscle test
   2. sensory test for light touch
   3. functional assessment for rolling in bed
   4. finger to nose

58. A physical therapist treats a client with Parkinson's disease. In order to improve the client's motor control, the therapist should incorporate which of the following techniques into the treatment session?

   1. alternating isometrics
   2. rhythmic initiation
   3. manual resisted exercise
   4. lumbar stabilization exercises in quadruped

59. A therapist examines a client diagnosed with cerebellar degeneration. Which of the following signs/symptoms is not characteristic of cerebellar degeneration?

   1. limb ataxia
   2. nystagmus
   3. dysmetria
   4. hypertonia

60. A therapist attempts to improve neck and upper back extension in an infant with developmental delay. When passively placed in prone prop, the infant quickly falls into the prone position. The therapist plans to position the child and then use toys and play objects to get the child to look up. Which position would be the most appropriate to meet the therapist's treatment objective?

    1. prone prop
    2. prone over a gymnastic ball
    3. prone over a wedge
    4. quadruped

61. An eleven month old child with cerebral palsy attempts to maintain a quadruped position. Which reflex would interfere with this activity if it did not integrate appropriately?

    1. Gallant reflex
    2. symmetrical tonic neck reflex
    3. plantar grasp reflex
    4. positive support reflex

62. A male therapist is treating a 16 year old female for a low back strain. During the treatment session the client makes several sexually suggestive remarks. The therapist ignores the remarks, but the client reiterates them during the next treatment session. The most appropriate therapist action is to _____?

    1. continue to ignore the client's remarks
    2. explain to the client that her remarks are offensive
    3. document the client's behavior in the medical record
    4. transfer the client to another therapist's schedule

63. A therapist attempts to schedule a client for an additional therapy session after completing the initial examination. The physician referral indicates the client is to be seen two times a week. The therapist suggests several possible times to the client, but the client insists she can only come in on Wednesday at 4:30. The therapist would like to accommodate the client, but already has two clients scheduled at that time. The most appropriate action is to _____?

    1. schedule the client on Wednesday at 4:30
    2. attempt to move one of the client's scheduled on Wednesday at 4:30 to a different time
    3. schedule the client with another therapist on Wednesday at 4:30
    4. inform the referring physician the client only will be seen once this week in therapy

64. A therapist develops a series of long and short term goals for a client. Which of the following is not a necessary component of a properly written goal?

    1. audience   + condition
    2. degree
    3. behavior
    4. priority

125

65. A physical therapist consults with an orthotist regarding the need for an ankle-foot orthosis for a stroke client. The client has difficulty moving from sitting to standing when wearing a prefabricated ankle-foot orthosis. The therapist indicates the client has poor strength at the ankle, intact sensation and does not have any edema or tonal influence. The most appropriate type of ankle-foot orthosis for the client would incorporate _____?

  1. an articulation at the ankle joint
  2. tone reducing features
  3. metal uprights
  4. dorsiflexion assist spring

66. A therapist establishes safe exercise intensity parameters for a phase I inpatient cardiac rehabilitation program. Which parameter would be the most appropriate for the phase I program?

  1. a maximum heart rate increase of 20 beats per minute above resting
  2. a maximum heart rate increase of 30 beats per minute above resting
  3. a maximum heart rate increase of 40 beats per minute above resting
  4. a maximum heart rate increase of 50 beats per minute above resting

67. A therapist provides preoperative instruction for a client scheduled for anterior cruciate ligament reconstructive surgery. During the treatment session, the client expresses to the therapist a sincere fear of dying during surgery. The therapist's most appropriate response would be _____?

  1. This surgery is done many times every day.
  2. I have never had a client of mine die yet.
  3. Surgery can be a very frightening thought.
  4. You will be back to athletics before you know it.

68. Premature ventricular contractions are the most commonly observed form of arrhythmias. Which of the following does not assist in precipitating PVCs?

  1. anxiety
  2. tobacco
  3. alcohol
  4. sodium

69. A therapist using an electrical stimulation device attempts to quantify several characteristics of a monophasic waveform. When measuring phase charge, the standard unit of measure is _____?

  1. coulomb
  2. ampere
  3. ohm
  4. seconds

70. A therapist instructs a client in ambulation activities using axillary crutches. What two points of control should be used when guarding the client?

    1. the client's thorax and hip
    2. the client's shoulder and hip
    3. the client's shoulder and thorax
    4. the client's elbow and hip

71. There can be many adverse effects when clients are fit incorrectly for a wheelchair. Which of the following could result from a wheelchair with excessive seat depth?

    1. decreased trunk stability
    2. increased weightbearing on the ischial tuberosities
    3. decreased balance
    4. increased pressure in the popliteal area

72. A therapist assesses the functional strength of a client's hip extensors while observing a client move from standing to sitting. What type of contraction occurs in the hip extensors during this activity?

    1. concentric
    2. eccentric
    3. isometric
    4. isotonic

73. A rehabilitation manager develops a quality assurance program that examines the extent to which physical therapists conform to accepted professional practices. This type of quality assurance program is most concerned with _____?

    1. structure
    2. process
    3. outcome
    4. product

74. A client referred to physical therapy with chronic low back pain has failed to make any progress toward meeting established goals in over three weeks of treatment. The therapist has employed a variety of treatment techniques, but has yet to observe any sign of subjective or objective improvement in the client's condition. The most appropriate action would be to _____?

    1. transfer the client to another therapist's schedule
    2. re-examine the client and establish new goals
    3. continue to modify the client's treatment plan
    4. alert the referring physician of the client's status

75. A client with cardiopulmonary pathology is referred to physical therapy. The therapist documents the following clinical signs: pallor, cyanosis, and skin coolness. These clinical signs are most consistent with _____?

1. cor pulmonale
2. anemia
3. atelectasis
4. diaphoresis

76. A physician instructs a client to take nonprescription or over the counter medication as part of his treatment program. Which of the following statements about over the counter medication is not accurate?

1. The Food and Drug Administration classifies drugs as prescription or nonprescription.
2. Over the counter medications are available without a prescription and can be purchased directly by consumers.
3. Over the counter medications usually contain low doses of their active ingredient.
4. Potentially harmful effects are not possible with over the counter medications.

77. A pregnant client in her third trimester completes a series of exercises in supine. In order to prevent vena cava compression during the exercise session the therapist should _____?

1. place a folded towel under the right side of the client's pelvis
2. place a folded towel under the left side of the client's pelvis
3. complete the exercises in sidelying
4. elevate the client's feet 12 inches

78. A therapist completes an upper extremity manual muscle test on a client diagnosed with rotator cuff tendonitis. Assuming the client has the ability to move the upper extremities against gravity, which of the following muscles would not be tested with the client in a supine position?

1. pronator teres
2. pectoralis major
3. lateral rotators of the shoulder
4. middle trapezius

79. A physical therapist is working with a child who has cerebral palsy with spastic diplegia. All of the following could be used to improve the child's ability to ambulate except _____?

1. stretching and range of motion
2. strengthening of underlying weak muscles
3. bilateral lower extremity activities such as "bunny hopping"
4. trunk and pelvis dissociation activities

80. A two year old with T10 spina bifida receives physical therapy for gait training. The preferred method when first teaching the child how to maintain standing is with the use of _____?

    1. bilateral HKAFOs and forearm crutches
    2. a parapodium and the parallel bars
    3. bilateral KAFOs and the parallel bars
    4. bilateral AFOs and the parallel bars

81. A physical therapist instructs the parents of a premature infant on proper positioning. The physical therapist should educate the parents to avoid _____ when placing their infant in supine?

    1. lower extremity extension
    2. slight neck flexion
    3. hands towards midline
    4. scapular protraction

82. A 45 year old female with psoriasis is referred to physical therapy. The client has several lesions on the posterior portion of the thigh extending into the popliteal fossa. The most appropriate therapeutic modality to treat the client's condition is _____?

    1. iontophoresis
    2. moist heat
    3. ultrasound
    4. ultraviolet

83. A therapist reviews a technical manual for an electrical stimulation unit. The manual discusses several inherent electrical terms such as voltage, current and resistance. Which of the following terms is commonly used to express current?

    1. ampere
    2. coulomb
    3. kilohm
    4. megohm

84. A client files suit against a physical therapist claiming that she was injured as a result of a specific treatment technique. In legal proceedings, which of the following would have the most impact on what actually happened at the time of the alleged negligent act?

    1. the client's recollections
    2. the therapist's recollections
    3. the referring physician's initial examination
    4. the physical therapist's daily documentation

85. A therapist instructs a client to ascend stairs using axillary crutches. Which of the following statements most accurately reflects proper guarding technique?

1. the therapist is positioned posterior and lateral on the affected side behind the client
2. the therapist is positioned anterior and lateral on the affected side in front of the client
3. the therapist is positioned posterior and lateral on the nonaffected side behind the client
4. the therapist is positioned anterior and lateral on the nonaffected side behind the client

86. A physical therapist prepares a client education program for an individual with chronic venous insufficiency. Which of the following would not be appropriate to include in the client education program?

1. wear shoes that accommodate to the size and shape of your feet
2. observe your skin daily for breakdown
3. wear your compression stockings only at night
4. keep your feet elevated as much as possible throughout the day

87. A 72 year old female six weeks status post stroke is scheduled for discharge from the hospital in one week. At the present time the client is unable to ambulate and requires maximal assistance to complete most transfers. Prior to her hospital admission the client lived alone in an apartment on the first floor. The most appropriate discharge plan would be _____?

1. home with no support services
2. a nursing home
3. home with physical therapy three times per week
4. home with a home health aide during the day

88. A therapist instructs a client in breathing exercises to improve ventilation and oxygenation. The therapist's treatment objective emphasizes the expansion of a selected area of the chest wall during inspiration. The most appropriate breathing exercise to achieve the desired outcome is _____?

1. deep breathing
2. diaphragmatic breathing
3. segmental breathing
4. abdominal breathing

89. A graded exercise test is performed on a client with pulmonary disease. During the test the therapist identifies that the client's systolic blood pressure has decreased by 20 mmHg. The most appropriate action is to _____?

1. continue the graded exercise test
2. discontinue the graded exercise test
3. assess the client's respiration rate
4. assess the client's forced expiratory volume in one second

90. A 16 year old complete C5 spinal cord injured client is two weeks status post injury. The client presently tolerates only 30 degrees on the tilt table secondary to orthostatic hypotension. Which transfer would be the most appropriate to utilize when moving the client from bed to the tilt table?

    1. hydraulic lift
    2. sliding transfer with draw sheet
    3. two person lift
    4. dependent standing pivot transfer

91. It is essential to maintain a sterile field once it has been established. Which of the following activities would not be in violation of a sterile field?

    1. sneezing while standing in front of a sterile field
    2. reaching across a sterile field
    3. turning your back to the field
    4. allowing a sterile object to touch another sterile object

92. Residual limb wrapping is often a necessary component of a treatment program following lower extremity amputation. Which of the following is not characteristic of a properly applied bandage?

    1. smooth and wrinkle free
    2. emphasizes angular turns
    3. provides pressure distally
    4. encourages proximal joint flexion

93. A therapist determines that a client rehabilitating from ankle surgery has consistent difficulty with functional activities that emphasize the frontal plane. Which of the following activities would be the most difficult for the client?

    1. anterior lunge
    2. 6 inch lateral step down
    3. 6 inch posterior step up
    4. 8 inch posterior step down

94. A client rehabilitating from a radial head fracture is examined in physical therapy. During the examination, the therapist notes that the client appears to have an elbow flexion contracture. Which of the following would not act as an appropriate active exercise technique to increase range of motion?

    1. contract relax
    2. hold relax
    3. maintained pressure
    4. rhythmic stabilization

95. A therapist monitors a client's pulse after ambulation activities. The therapist notes that at times the rhythm of the pulse is irregular. When assessing the client's pulse rate, the therapist should measure the clients pulse for _____ seconds?

1. 10
2. 15
3. 30
4. 60

96. A therapist adjusts the height of the parallel bars in preparation for client ambulation. When at the appropriate height, the parallel bars should provide _____?

1. 5 - 15 degrees of elbow flexion
2. 15 - 25 degrees of elbow flexion
3. 30 - 40 degrees of elbow flexion
4. 35 - 45 degrees of elbow flexion

97. Standard postural drainage positions for specific lung segments utilize a variety of client positions, including sitting, sidelying, supine, and prone. Postural drainage of the _____ typically is administered with the client in sitting?

1. anterior basal segments of the lower lobes
2. posterior segments of the upper lobes
3. posterior basal segments of the lower lobes
4. right middle lobe

98. When evaluating a client for a wheelchair, a therapist determines that the client's hip width in sitting and the measurement from the back of the buttocks to the popliteal space are each 16 inches. Given these measurements, which of the following wheelchair sizes would best fit this client?

1. seat width 16 inches, seat depth 14 inches
2. seat width 18 inches, seat depth 18 inches
3. seat width 16 inches, seat depth 18 inches
4. seat width 18 inches, seat depth 14 inches

99. A client recently admitted to the hospital with an acute illness is referred to physical therapy. During a scheduled treatment session the client asks what effect anemia will have on his ability to complete a formal exercise program. The most appropriate therapist response is?

1. you may feel as though your muscles are weak
2. you may experience frequent nausea
3. your aerobic capacity may be reduced
4. you may have a tendency to become fatigued

100. When performing range of motion exercises with a client who suffered a head injury, a physical therapist notes that the client lacks full elbow extension and classifies the end feel as hard. The most likely cause is _____?

    1. heterotopic ossification
    2. spasticity of the biceps
    3. anterior capsular tightness
    4. triceps weakness

101. A client rehabilitating from injuries sustained in a motor vehicle accident is referred to physical therapy for gait training with an appropriate assistive device. The therapist attempts to instruct the client using axillary crutches, but feels the assistive device does not offer the client enough stability or support. Which of the following assistive devices would be the most appropriate for the client?

    1. walker
    2. cane
    3. Lofstrand crutches
    4. parallel bars

102. A therapist attempts to develop a problem list after examining a client with a transtibial amputation. Which of the following would be the most appropriate entry in the client problem list?

    1. donning and doffing prosthesis requires verbal cues
    2. donning and doffing prosthesis requires verbal cues and minimal assist of 1
    3. dependence with donning and doffing prosthesis
    4. independent donning and doffing prosthesis in one week

103. The director of rehabilitation in an orthopedic private practice prepares a list of interview questions for applicants applying for a vacant position. Which of the following would be an acceptable interview question?

    1. Are you in good health?
    2. How much weight can you lift?
    3. Have you held a position like this in the past?
    4. Have you ever filed a workers' compensation claim?

104. A 42 year old female who is unable to satisfactorily control the retention and release of urine uses a catheter. Which type of urinary catheter would not be appropriate for the client?

    1. indwelling urinary catheter
    2. external urinary catheter
    3. Foley catheter
    4. suprapubic catheter

105. A client ambulating with an IV in place should be instructed to grasp the IV pole at what level?

    1. a level where the infusion site is above heart level
    2. a level where the infusion site is at heart level
    3. a level where the infusion site is below heart level
    4. a client with an IV in place should not participate in ambulation activities

106. A therapist monitors a 6 foot 3 inch, 275 pound, male's blood pressure using the brachial artery. Which of the following is most important when selecting an appropriate size blood pressure cuff?

    1. client age
    2. percent body fat
    3. somatotype
    4. extremity circumference

107. Accurate, clear, and concise documentation is becoming increasingly important for all health care providers. Which of the following suggestions to improve documentation would not be useful?

    1. avoid empty or open lines between entries in the medical record
    2. make sure all entries in the medical record are typewritten
    3. use abbreviations that have been standardized or accepted by a specific facility or the profession
    4. co-sign the entries of other medical personnel when necessary according to state and facility requirements

108. A client informs his therapist that he has to use the bathroom immediately after being transported outside the hospital to practice car transfers. The therapist's most appropriate response to meet the client's physical need is to _____?

    1. ask the client if it is an emergency
    2. complete the transfer training as quickly as possible and allow the client to use the bathroom
    3. transport the client back into the hospital to use the bathroom
    4. instruct the client that in the future he should use the bathroom before beginning physical therapy

109. A therapist examines a client seven days status post total hip replacement. The client's medical record indicates the surgeon utilized an anterolateral surgical approach. Which of the following motions would be the most important to restrict during the initial phase of rehabilitation?

    1. knee extension
    2. knee flexion
    3. hip external rotation
    4. hip internal rotation

110. A therapist monitors a client's pulse rate using the radial artery. Which of the following general statements regarding pulse rate is not accurate?

    1. pulse rate is increased with physical exertion
    2. pulse rate is decreased during relaxation or sleep
    3. pulse rate is decreased with anxiety or stress
    4. pulse rate is higher in children than adults

111. A client informs her therapist how frustrated she feels after being examined by her physician. The client explains that she becomes so nervous, she can not ask any questions during scheduled office visits. The therapist's most appropriate response is to _____?

    1. offer to go with the client to her next scheduled physician visit
    2. offer to call the physician and ask any relevant questions
    3. suggest that the client write down questions for the physician and bring them with her to the next scheduled visit
    4. tell the client it is a very normal response to be nervous in the presence of a physician

112. A physical therapist observes an electrocardiogram of a client on beta-blockers. Which of the following ECG changes could be facilitated by the beta-blockers?

    1. bradycardia
    2. tachycardia
    3. increased AV conduction time
    4. ST segment sagging

113. A therapist instructs a client with acute Achilles tendonitis in a home exercise program. As part of the program, the therapist attempts to reduce the inflammation in the involved region. Which of the following modalities would be the most beneficial to achieve the therapist's goal?

    1. continuous ultrasound
    2. pulsed ultrasound
    3. ice massage
    4. whirlpool

114. An athlete is forced to contemplate knee surgery after spraining the anterior cruciate ligament while playing soccer. Which situation would provide the most direct support for an anterior cruciate ligament reconstruction?

    1. grade III ACL and grade I PCL injury
    2. grade III ACL sprain with lateral meniscal involvement
    3. grade II ACL sprain with medial meniscal involvement
    4. functional instability

115. A therapist asks a client who has been inconsistent with his attendance in physical therapy, why he is having difficulty keeping scheduled appointments. The client responds that it is difficult to understand the scheduling card that lists the appointments. The therapist's most appropriate action would be to _____?

    1. contact the referring physician to discuss the client's poor attendance in therapy
    2. make sure the client is given a scheduling card at the conclusion of each session
    3. write down the client's appointments on a piece of paper in a manner that the client can understand
    4. discharge the client from physical therapy

116. A client status post coronary artery bypass graft is exercising in a phase I cardiac rehabilitation program. While exercising, the client's pulse rate is measured as 125 beats/minute and her respiration rate is 32 breaths/minute. Based on the client's vital signs, the therapist's most immediate response should be to _____?

    1. stop the exercise session and continue to monitor the client's vital signs
    2. continue with the exercise session and continue to monitor the client's vital signs
    3. notify the referring physician of the client's vital signs
    4. document the client's response to exercise in the medical record

117. A therapist reviews the medical chart of a client diagnosed with a fracture of the lower thoracic spine. The chart indicates the client has worn an anterior control thoracolumbar-sacral-orthosis for eight weeks. What is the primary purpose of the anterior control TLSO? Jewett brace

    1. prevent thoracic flexion
    2. prevent thoracic extension
    3. prevent lumbar flexion
    4. prevent lumbar extension

118. Which of the following can be used to examine and objectively document motor return in a client with hemiplegia?

    1. Tinetti Balance and Gait Assessment Scale
    2. Somatosensory Organization Test
    3. Functional Independence Measure
    4. Fugl-Meyer Assessment of Motor Performance

119. A therapist palpates proximally along the lateral border of the fifth metatarsal of a client's foot. Which bone would be palpable as the therapist continues to palpate proximally along the lateral border of the foot?

    1. cuboid
    2. second cuneiform
    3. third cuneiform
    4. navicular

120. A therapist establishes the following short term goal for a client rehabilitating from total knee replacement surgery: Client will ambulate with walker 50% weightbearing and moderate assist of 1 for 20 feet within one week. Three days later, the client successfully achieves the established goal. Which of the following would be the most appropriate revision of the short term goal?

1. ambulate with walker 25% WB and moderate assist of 1 for 25 feet within one week
2. ambulate with walker 50% WB and moderate assist of 2 for 30 feet within one week
3. ambulate with walker 50% WB and minimal assist of 1 for 30 feet within one week
4. ambulate with the walker 25% WB and minimal assist of 1 for 10 feet within one week

121. Clients who are unable to meet their daily nutritional needs independently often require the use of a feeding device. A feeding device such as a nasogastric tube can be utilized for a variety of purposes. Which of the following does not accurately describe a potential use of the nasogastric tube?

1. administer medications directly into the gastrointestinal tract
2. obtain gastric specimens
3. remove fluid or gas from the stomach
4. obtain venous blood samples

122. All ambulation aids provide varying amounts of stability and support. Many of the aids also have distinct disadvantages, usually resulting from the shape and configuration of the device. Which of the following ambulation aids most likely would cause injury to axillary vessels and nerves when used improperly?

1. walker
2. axillary crutches
3. Lofstrand crutches
4. parallel bars

123. A therapist conducts a goniometric assessment of the wrist and hand. When determining the available range of motion for thumb flexion, the therapist should align the axis of the goniometer over the _____?

1. dorsal aspect of the first carpometacarpal joint
2. palmar aspect of the first carpometacarpal joint
3. midway between the dorsal aspect of the first and second carpometacarpal joints
4. midway between the palmar aspect of the first and second carpometacarpal joints

124. A therapist examines a client status post amputation. Which amputation level would be most susceptible to a hip flexion contracture?

1. transfemoral
2. knee disarticulate
3. long transtibial
4. short transtibial

125. A therapist examines a client with post-polio syndrome. Given the client's diagnosis, which of the following is the least important component of the examination?

   1. strength
   2. sensation
   3. endurance
   4. functional mobility

126. When observing a client ambulating, a therapist notes that the client's gait has the following characteristics: narrow base of support, short step length bilaterally, and decreased trunk rotation. This gait pattern is often observed in clients with a diagnosis of _____?

   1. stroke
   2. Parkinson's disease
   3. post-polio syndrome
   4. multiple sclerosis

127. A therapist attempts to assess a client's fine motor coordination following wrist surgery. Which of the following tasks would require the greatest fine motor coordination?

   1. stacking large blocks
   2. assembling small pins, collars and washers
   3. turning cards
   4. picking up large heavy objects

128. A variety of factors can influence blood pressure. Which individual would you expect to have the lowest systolic blood pressure?

   1. 10 year old
   2. 30 year old
   3. 50 year old
   4. 70 year old

129. A therapist designs a cardiovascular training program for a 29 year old male rehabilitating from a lower extremity injury. The client has no known cardiovascular pathology and has been cleared for exercise by his physician. The client's maximum heart rate during exercise should be calculated as _____?

   1. 170 beats per minute
   2. 180 beats per minute
   3. 191 beats per minute
   4. 201 beats per minute

130. Physical therapy aides can play an important role in the daily operation of a physical therapy department. Which of the following activities would not be appropriate for an aide to perform?

    1. cleaning and maintaining exercise equipment
    2. transporting clients
    3. preparing a treatment area
    4. implementing an exercise program

131. A therapist prepares to complete an assisted standing pivot transfer with a client that requires moderate assistance. In order to increase a client's independence with the transfer, which of the following instructions would be the most appropriate?

    1. I want you to help me perform the transfer.
    2. Try to utilize your own strength to complete the transfer.
    3. Only grab onto me if it is absolutely necessary.
    4. Use the power in your legs to assist you during the transfer.

132. A therapist assesses the ligamentous integrity of a client's knee by completing a series of special tests. The most accurate way to determine if the client's ligamentous integrity is compromised is to _____?

    1. compare the millimeters of ligamentous laxity to established norms
    2. instruct the referring physician to order radiographs
    3. compare the ligamentous laxity in the involved knee to the uninvolved knee
    4. compare the ligamentous laxity to other clients in the clinic without knee pathology

133. A therapist examines a 48 year old male with degenerative joint disease. The referring physician indicates that the client should be seen in physical therapy three times per week. During the examination the client indicates that the car ride to therapy takes approximately 50 minutes and that child care duties make frequent physical therapy visits impossible. The therapist's most appropriate action is to _____?

    1. reduce the number of weekly visits and notify the referring physician.
    2. transfer the client to another therapist's schedule
    3. ask the client to discuss the matter with his physician
    4. treat the client three times per week

134. A therapist instructs a client with a lower extremity amputation to wrap her residual limb. Which of the following would be the least acceptable method of securing the bandages?

    1. clips — Dangerous
    2. safety pins — not as bad as clips
    3. tape
    4. velcro

135. A client uses transcutaneous electrical neuromuscular stimulation for pain modulation. Which set of parameters best describes conventional TENS?

    1. 50-100 pps, short phase duration, low intensity
    2. 100-150 pps, short phase duration, high intensity
    3. 150-200 pps, long phase duration, low intensity
    4. 200-250 pps, short phase duration, low intensity

136. A therapist observes a client's skin shortly after applying moist heat to the lower back. The therapist identifies several signs of heat intolerance including uneven blotching and a surface rash. The most appropriate action is to _____?

    1. continue with the present treatment
    2. select an alternate superficial heating agent
    3. limit moist heat exposure to five minutes
    4. discontinue the moist heat and document the findings

137. A therapist works with a client rehabilitating from a traumatic brain injury on a mat program. The program emphasizes various developmental positions to prepare a client for ambulation activities. Which developmental position would be the most demanding?

    1. hooklying
    2. quadruped
    3. kneeling
    4. modified plantigrade

138. A severely disabled client is referred to physical therapy for gait training. The client exhibits good balance and coordination and has normal upper extremity strength. The client currently is using a wheelchair for the majority of her transportation and occasionally uses a swing to gait pattern with Lofstrand crutches. The client reports being frustrated by the lack of speed using the swing to gait and would like to learn an alternate gait pattern. What gait pattern would be the most appropriate for the client?

    1. two point alternating
    2. three point
    3. four point alternating
    4. swing through

139. A therapist prepares a client status post stroke with global aphasia for discharge from a rehabilitation hospital. The client will be returning home with her husband and daughter. The most appropriate form of education to facilitate a safe discharge is to _____?

    1. perform hands on training sessions with the client and family members
    2. videotape the client performing transfers and ADLs
    3. provide written instructions on all ADLs and functional tasks
    4. meet with family members to discuss the client's present status and abilities

140. A therapist is required to transfer a 250 lb. dependent client from a mat table to a wheelchair. The therapist is concerned about her ability to independently transfer the client, but is unable to locate another staff member to offer assistance. The most appropriate action would be to _____?

1. instruct the client to take a more active role in the transfer
2. attempt to complete the transfer independently, but stop immediately if body mechanics are compromised
3. inform the nursing staff to complete the transfer
4. wait until another staff member is available to assist with the transfer

141. A client successfully completes ten anterior lunges. The therapist would like to modify the activity to maximally challenge the client in the sagittal plane. Which of the following modifications would be the most appropriate?

1. anterior lunge with concurrent bilateral elbow flexion to 45 degrees with five pound weights
2. anterior lunge with concurrent bilateral shoulder flexion to 90 degrees with five pound weights
3. anterior lunge with concurrent unilateral shoulder flexion to 90 degrees with a five pound weight
4. anterior lunge with concurrent bilateral shoulder abduction to 45 degrees with five pound weights

142. A therapist teaches a client positioned in supine to posteriorly rotate her pelvis. The client has full active and passive range of motion in the upper extremities, but is unable to achieve full shoulder flexion while maintaining the posterior pelvic tilt. Which of the following could best explain these findings?

1. capsular tightness
2. latissimus dorsi tightness
3. pectoralis minor tightness
4. quadratus lumborum tightness

143. A clinical instructor asks a student to complete three selected joint mobilization techniques on a client diagnosed with adhesive capsulitis. Which learning domain is emphasized with the desired task?

1. cognitive
2. psychomotor
3. affective
4. psychosocial

144. A client sustains a deep laceration on the right thigh after falling into a modality cart. The laceration causes immediate and excessive bleeding. The therapist should first _____?

1. apply direct pressure over the laceration
2. examine the lower extremity
3. put on gloves
4. contact the chief physical therapist

145. As part of an initial examination, a physical therapist develops long term goals for a client who has complete quadriplegia at the C5 level. All of the following are appropriate long term goals for this client except _____?

   1. complete lower extremity self range of motion in bed independently
   2. eat independently with adaptive equipment
   3. propel a manual wheelchair 15 feet on level surfaces independently
   4. direct a caretaker to perform a car transfer

146. A client with paraplegia is interested in learning how to perform a wheelie to assist with community mobility. The client is independent with basic wheelchair propulsion. When instructing the client to perform a wheelie, the therapist first should teach the client to _____?

   1. make small adjustments (forward and backward) after being placed in the wheelie position
   2. move into the wheelie position
   3. perform turns while holding the wheelie position
   4. statically hold the wheelie position after being placed in it by the therapist

147. Physical therapists and physical therapist assistants perform many of the same functions in the clinic. Which of the following activities would not be appropriate for a physical therapist assistant to perform?

   1. application of superficial modalities
   2. instruction of a client in gait training
   3. complete documentation in the medical record
   4. modification of an established plan of care

148. A client sustains a traction injury to the brachial plexus in a motor vehicle accident and has resultant C5 and C6 nerve root involvement. Which of the following muscles would be most affected by the injury?

   1. flexor carpi ulnaris
   2. levator scapulae
   3. pectoralis minor
   4. pectoralis major

149. A physical therapist observes a burn on the dorsal surface of a client's arm. The therapist notes that the wound appears to involve the epidermis and most of the dermis. The wound area is mottled red with a number of blisters. The therapist informs the client that healing should take place in less than three weeks. This description is most indicative of a _____?

   1. superficial burn
   2. superficial partial-thickness burn
   3. deep partial-thickness burn
   4. full-thickness burn

150. A group of physical therapists develop a research project which examines the effect of increased abdominal muscle strength on forced vital capacity and forced expiratory volume. In order to conduct the study, the therapists are required to have the approval of the Hospital Institutional Review Board. The primary purpose of the committee is to _____?

    1. protect the hospital from unnecessary litigation
    2. ensure that established client care standards are not compromised
    3. examine the design of the research project
    4. assess the financial ramifications of the research project

151. Members of a community health task force evaluate a proposal for a new adolescent screening program. Several members of the task force raise questions as to the validity of the screening instrument. Which measure of validity examines the instrument's ability to identify diseased persons by comparing true positives?

    1. adaptability
    2. selectivity
    3. sensitivity
    4. specificity

152. A client who has difficulty controlling the release and retention of urine uses a urinary catheter. Upon beginning to examine the client, the therapist notices that the collection bag is almost completely full. The most appropriate action is to _____?

    1. continue with the examination and periodically monitor the collection bag
    2. disconnect the collection bag during the examination
    3. empty the collection bag
    4. contact the client's nurse and request assistance

153. A therapist discusses the importance of proper skin care with a client and his family. Which of the following sites is least likely to develop a pressure ulcer in a wheelchair dependent client?

    1. scapula
    2. ischium
    3. heel
    4. elbow

154. A group of physical therapists conducts scoliosis screenings on adolescents as part of physical therapy week. The most appropriate action after identifying an adolescent with a moderate scoliotic curve is to _____?

    1. refer the adolescent for further orthopedic assessment
    2. educate the adolescent as to the causes of scoliosis
    3. devise an exercise program for the adolescent
    4. instruct the adolescent in the importance of proper posture

155. A therapist orders a wheelchair for a client recently admitted to a rehabilitation hospital. How many inches above the chair seat is the armrest on a standard adult wheelchair?

    1. 5 inches
    2. 7 inches
    3. 9 inches
    4. 11 inches

156. A therapist designs a treatment program for a client with a traumatic head injury. The client currently is classified as confused-agitated. Which of the following guidelines would be the least beneficial when developing the treatment program?

    1. The therapist should emphasize previously learned skills and avoid teaching only new skills.
    2. The therapist should maintain a calm and focused affect.
    3. The therapist should concentrate on one specific activity for each treatment session.
    4. The therapist should schedule the client at the same time and same place each day.

157. A therapist orders a wheelchair for a client with C7 complete quadriplegia. Which of the following wheelchairs would be the most appropriate for the client?

    1. electric wheelchair with chin controls
    2. manual wheelchair with handrim projections
    3. manual wheelchair with friction surface handrims
    4. manual wheelchair with standard handrims

158. A therapist checks the water temperature of the hot pack machine after several clients report the heat being very strong. Which of the following temperatures would be acceptable?

    1. 71 degrees Celsius
    2. 88 degrees Celsius
    3. 130 degrees Fahrenheit
    4. 190 degrees Fahrenheit

159. A physical therapy department plans a study to examine rehabilitation outcomes in clients who have undergone anterior cruciate ligament reconstruction. The study will include a sample of clients from 25 orthopedic surgeons in the local region. If the therapists compile a list of all eligible clients and select every third client to participate in the study, what type of sampling was used?

    1. simple random sampling
    2. stratified sampling
    3. systematic sampling
    4. cluster sampling

160. A therapist prepares to mobilize the glenohumeral joint by placing the joint in its resting position. Which of the following explanations best describes why this position is used commonly for joint mobilization?

  1. joint compressive forces are minimal in the resting position
  2. assessment manipulations are performed easily in the resting position
  3. there is maximal congruency in the articular surfaces in the resting position
  4. oscillations are performed easily in the resting position

161. A physical therapist designs a research study in which it is desirable to limit the risk when making a conclusion or inference from the study. Which of the following levels of significance would be the most appropriate for the study?

  1. .05
  2. .01
  3. 1.0
  4. 10

162. A client who has completed six months of therapy receives a referral for eight additional weeks of physical therapy. The therapist feels the client has plateaued and is not a realistic candidate for continued therapy. The therapist's most appropriate action is to _____?

  1. continue the client in physical therapy for eight additional weeks
  2. re-examine the client and develop new short and long term goals
  3. conduct a four week trial to determine if the client has made objective progress
  4. contact the referring physician and discuss the concerns regarding the client's rehabilitation potential

163. A therapist uses palpation to assess upper lobe expansion during quiet and deep breathing. Which of the following descriptions most accurately describes proper hand placement when palpating the upper lobe?

  1. place the palms firmly against the chest wall and hook the fingers over the posterior axillary fold
  2. place the palms of the hand firmly over the anterior aspect of the chest from the fourth rib cranially and hook the fingers around the trapezii
  3. place the thumbs over the spine of the scapulae so that the fingers reach around the anterolateral aspects of the neck
  4. extend the thumbs over the posterior midline of the back and hook the fingers around the anterior axillary fold

164. A therapist presents an inservice entitled, "Preventing Pressure Ulcers" to a group of physical therapy aides. As part of the inservice, the therapist identifies risk factors associated with the development of pressure ulcers. Which of the following would not be considered a significant risk factor?

    1. nutritional deficiencies
    2. incontinence
    3. psychological stress and depression
    4. vocational dysfunction

165. A client suffers a chemical burn on the cubital area of the elbow. Which position would be the most appropriate for splinting of the involved upper extremity?

    1. elbow flexion and forearm pronation
    2. elbow flexion and forearm supination
    3. elbow extension and forearm pronation
    4. elbow extension and forearm supination

166. Electromyography is performed on a client to objectively determine the extent of pathology after sustaining a brachial plexus injury. Which of the following responses is most indicative of a normal muscle at rest?

    1. electrical silence
    2. spontaneous potentials
    3. polyphasic potentials
    4. occasional motor unit potentials

167. A client with a C7 nerve root injury is examined in physical therapy. Which of the following objective findings would be most indicative of C7 involvement?

    1. paresthesia over the little finger
    2. weak triceps and wrist flexor muscles
    3. paresthesia over the thumb
    4. weak biceps and supinator muscles

168. A physical therapist examines a client diagnosed with acromioclavicular joint dysfunction. The therapist instructs the client to abduct his arm in a coronal plane to 180 degrees. Which portion of the range of motion would you most expect to elicit pain in the acromioclavicular joint?

    1. 30-70 degrees
    2. 50-90 degrees
    3. 90-120 degrees
    4. 120-180 degrees

169. A physical therapist employed in a skilled nursing facility frequently treats cognitively impaired elderly clients. Which of the following guidelines is not recommended when working with this particular population?

1. encourage the use of hands on treatment
2. explain frequently, consistently, and repetitively when necessary
3. change the client's environment and staff frequently
4. simplify commands and label items for easy recognition

170. A therapist completes a quantitative gait analysis on a client rehabilitating from a lower extremity injury. As part of the examination the therapist measures the number of steps taken by the client in a 30 second period. This measurement technique can be used to measure _____?

1. acceleration
2. cadence
3. velocity
4. speed

171. Members of a health promotion task force design a program that annually will screen individuals in selected retirement communities for osteoporosis. Which screening tool would be the most cost effective and reliable to incorporate as part of the program?

1. physical activity survey
2. dietary analysis
3. measuring height
4. urinalysis screening

172. A cardiac client undergoes a low-level symptom limited exercise treadmill test that begins at 1.5 METs and progresses to 4 METs. Which of the following activities would require an energy expenditure of approximately 4 METs?

1. sitting quietly at rest
2. level walking at 1 mph
3. level walking at 3 mph
4. level walking at 5 mph

173. A physical therapist prepares a client for prosthetic training. Which of the following amputations would require the highest energy expenditure when using the appropriate prosthesis?

1. bilateral transtibial amputations
2. unilateral transtibial amputation
3. unilateral transfemoral amputation
4. Syme's amputation

174. A client rehabilitating from a total hip replacement is scheduled for home physical therapy. The therapist assigned to the case attempts to schedule the client, but the client indicates that she will be unavailable for the next week due to a death in the family. The most appropriate therapist action is to _____?

1. insist that the client participate in physical therapy
2. discharge the client secondary to noncompliance
3. document the conversation with the client and notify the physician
4. ask the physician to convince the client to begin physical therapy immediately

175. A therapist positions a client in prone with the knee flexed to 70 degrees prior to completing a manual muscle test of the hamstrings. To isolate the biceps femoris the therapist should _____?

1. place the thigh in slight lateral rotation and the leg in slight lateral rotation on the thigh
2. place the thigh in slight medial rotation and the leg in slight medial rotation on the thigh
3. position the knee in 100 degrees of flexion
4. position the knee in 120 degrees of flexion

176. A therapist reviews a client's blood gas analysis. The therapist identifies that the $Paco_2$ is elevated and the pH is below the normal level. These findings are most representative of _____?

1. respiratory acidosis
2. respiratory alkalosis
3. metabolic acidosis
4. metabolic alkalosis

177. A therapist strongly suspects a client is intoxicated after arriving for his treatment session. When asked if he has been drinking, the client indicates he consumed six or seven alcoholic beverages before driving to therapy. The therapist's most appropriate action is to _____?

1. continue to treat the client, assuming he can remain inoffensive to other clients
2. modify the client's present treatment program to minimize the effects of alcohol
3. contact a member of the client's family to take the client home
4. instruct the client to leave the clinic

178. A therapist instructs a client to complete a biceps strengthening exercise using a ten pound dumbbell in standing. The exercise requires the client to maximally flex her elbow twelve times without moving the trunk. While observing the client performing the exercise, it becomes apparent that the client is unable to maintain her trunk in a stationary position. Which of the following modifications would be the most appropriate?

1. decrease the number of repetitions to six
2. decrease the dumbbell weight to five pounds
3. instruct the client to perform the exercise while sitting on a stool
4. no modifications are necessary

179. A therapist prepares to apply a sterile dressing to a wound after debridement. The therapist begins the process by drying the wound using a towel. The therapist applies medication to the wound using a gauze pad and then applies a series of dressings which are secured using a bandage. Application of the _____ would not require the use of sterile technique?

1. bandage
2. dressings
3. medication
4. towel

180. A therapist interviews a client in an attempt to gather information to assist with discharge planning. The client is rehabilitating from an intertrochanteric fracture sustained six weeks ago after a fall. The client has moderate dementia, but has no other significant past medical history. Which of the following situations would present the client with the largest barrier toward living independently?

1. The client resides alone and has no outside support from family or friends.
2. The client is no longer able to drive and relies on a neighbor for all cooking, cleaning, and shopping.
3. The client has a two story home.
4. The client resides with a woman who has rheumatoid arthritis.

181. A therapist examines a client diagnosed with Guillain-Barre syndrome. All of the following are signs/symptoms associated with this syndrome except _____?

1. difficulty breathing
2. areflexia
3. weakness
4. absent sensation

182. A physical therapist examines a 42 year old self referred female. The client describes the onset of a variety of medical problems approximately one month ago. The client's reported problems include right lower extremity weakness, decreased balance and blurred vision. The physical therapy examination confirms the client's complaints, in addition to identifying decreased pinprick sensation and ankle clonus in the right lower extremity. The suspected diagnosis of this client is _____?

1. diabetes
2. multiple sclerosis
3. stroke
4. Parkinson's disease

183. A 78 year old male, one month status post open reduction and internal fixation of an intertrochanteric fracture is referred to physical therapy. The client has pain with active movement and decreased hip range of motion. Which of the following modalities would be contraindicated for the client?

1. moist heat
2. pulsed ultrasound
3. cryotherapy
4. shortwave diathermy

184. A physical therapist performs a wheelchair evaluation for a client with multiple sclerosis. The client recently fell while ambulating and sustained a fracture of the right tibia. Since the client is presently unable to bear weight through the involved extremity, the client has difficulty transferring from a chair to a bed. Which of the following wheelchair prescriptions is most appropriate for the client?

1. light weight wheelchair, removable armrests, removable elevating leg rests
2. light weight wheelchair, removable armrests, nonremovable leg rests
3. light weight wheelchair, nonremovable armrests, removable elevating leg rests
4. standard wheelchair, nonremovable armrests, and leg rests

185. A therapist positions a client in sidelying and performs a talar tilt test. A positive talar tilt test would be most indicative of a _____?

1. calcaneofibular ligament injury
2. ligamentous instability
3. deltoid ligament injury
4. excessive tibial torsion

186. A physical therapist treats a client who is status post traumatic brain injury. The client is classified as level four on the Ranchos Los Amigos Level of Cognitive Functioning Scale. Which of the following would be the least appropriate to include in the client's physical therapy session?

1. redirection to tasks
2. random practice, using a variety of tasks
3. repetition of instructions
4. ambulation in busy environments

187. According to the Motor Control / Task Oriented Approach, a physical therapy treatment session always should include _____?

1. tone reducing activities
2. positioning
3. functional activities
4. developmental positions

188. A therapist completes a daily progress note utilizing a S.O.A.P. format. Which of the following entries would not belong in the objective section?

1. will receive continuous ultrasound to the right anterior shoulder at 1.5 W/cm^2 for 5 minutes
2. incision on the left anterior forearm covered with steri-strips
3. left lower extremity range of motion within normal limits
4. tenderness to palpation in L1-L2 area

189. A physical therapist is treating a client with Parkinson's disease. The client has trouble initiating movement and is unable to ambulate independently. The client reports that he has fallen on three separate occasions within the last two months while attempting to ambulate. Which assistive device would be the most appropriate for this client?

1. rolling walker
2. walker
3. axillary crutches
4. small base quad cane

190. A client with muscle weakness and compromised balance uses a four-point gait pattern with two canes. When ascending stairs the most practical method is to _____?

1. use the handrail with the right hand and place the two canes in the left hand
2. use the handrail with the left hand and place the two canes in the right hand
3. place one cane in each hand and avoid using the handrail
4. place the two canes in the left hand and avoid using the handrail

191. A physical therapist receives a referral for a client who is one week status post head injury. In the client's medical record it notes that the client demonstrates decorticate posturing. This type of posturing is characterized by _____?

    1. upper extremity extension and lower extremity flexion
    2. upper extremity flexion and lower extremity flexion
    3. upper extremity extension and lower extremity extension
    4. upper extremity flexion and lower extremity extension

192. A twelve month old child with cerebral palsy demonstrates an abnormal persistence of the positive support reflex. During therapy this would most likely interfere with _____?

    1. sitting activities
    2. standing activities
    3. prone on elbows activities
    4. supine activities

193. A physical therapist treats a client with limited shoulder range of motion. The therapist feels that the client's range of motion limitation is due to pain and not a specific tissue restriction. Which mobilization grade would be most appropriate to treat this client?

    1. Grade I, II
    2. Grade II, III
    3. Grade III, IV
    4. Grade IV, V

194. A therapist assesses the hip range of motion of a client with excessive anteversion. Which of the following clinical findings is common in a client with anteversion?

    1. increased hip lateral rotation and decreased medial rotation
    2. increased hip medial rotation and decreased lateral rotation
    3. increased hip abduction and decreased adduction
    4. increased hip flexion and decreased extension

195. A client diagnosed with lateral epicondylitis is referred to physical therapy. The therapist elects to use iontophoresis over the lateral epicondyle. Which type of current would the therapist use to administer the treatment?

    1. direct
    2. alternating
    3. pulsatile
    4. interferential

196. A client with hemiplegia is ambulating with an ankle-foot orthosis. The therapist notes that the client's involved foot frequently drags during the initial swing phase of gait. To treat this problem most effectively the therapist should emphasize _____?

    1. eccentric strengthening of the hamstrings
    2. eccentric strengthening of the gluteus medius
    3. concentric strengthening of the plantar flexors
    4. concentric strengthening of the iliopsoas/rectus femoris

197. A physical therapist uses the upper extremity D1, E proprioceptive neuromuscular facilitation pattern and is resisting elbow extension with the goal of increasing the client's ability to extend her wrist. This is an example of _____?

    1. reciprocal excitation
    2. successive induction
    3. irradiation
    4. quick stretch

198. A client who has suffered a stroke four weeks ago is beginning to show the ability to produce movement patterns not dictated solely by limb synergies. According to Brunnstrom, this client is in which stage of recovery?

    1. two
    2. three
    3. four
    4. six

199. A therapist works with a client to improve bed mobility. Which of the following techniques will most effectively increase the client's hip stability?

    1. lower trunk rotation in the hooklying position
    2. bridging
    3. assisted hip and knee flexion in supine
    4. hip abduction and adduction in the hooklying position

200. A therapist completes a posture screening and a gross range of motion examination on a client referred to therapy with patella tendonitis. The therapist determines that the client has extremely limited lower extremity flexibility, most notably in her hip flexors. What common structural deformity often is associated with tight hip flexors?

    1. scoliosis
    2. kyphosis
    3. lordosis
    4. spondylosis

Answer Key

1. Answer: 1   Resource: Minor (309)

    When ascending a curb a client should lead with the uninvolved lower extremity in order
    to avoid placing unnecessary force on the involved extremity.

2. Answer: 2   Resource: Pierson (133)

    A hydraulic lift can be a safe and efficient mode to transfer large or dependent clients with
    little physical exertion.

3. Answer: 2   Resource: Magee (188)

    Passive shoulder complex flexion is approximately 180 degrees, however glenohumeral
    abduction is 120 degrees with approximately 60 degrees of motion occurring at the
    scapulothoracic joint.

4. Answer: 1   Resource: Kendall (147)

    Sway-back is synonymous with excessive lordosis. Individuals with weakness of the
    abdominal muscles often present with an anterior pelvic tilt and thus a lordotic posture.

5. Answer: 4   Resource: Pierson (61)

    As the intensity of exercise plateaus, a client will accommodate to the level of exercise
    and his/her respiration rate will tend to decrease.

6. Answer: 1   Resource: Brannon (50)

    Vital capacity is defined as the amount of air that can be exhaled following a maximal
    inspiratory effort. Vital capacity varies directly with height and indirectly with age.

7. Answer: 1   Resource: Kendall (385)

    The infraspinatus muscle is innervated by the suprascapular nerve (C4, C5, C6) which
    extends from the superior trunk of the brachial plexus.

8. Answer: 3   Resource: Paz (616)

    Repositioning the bedrail is an immediate and appropriate response that is within the
    therapist's scope of practice.

9. Answer: 2   Resource: Minor (39)

    An acceptable target heart rate during cardiovascular exercise is between .6 -.8 of the age
    predicted maximal heart rate.

10. Answer: 4   Resource: Minor (54)

    Once a nonsterile object is placed within a sterile field, the entire sterile field should be
    considered nonsterile.

11. Answer: 3   Resource: Norkin and White (26)

Although the client can flex his right shoulder to 173 degrees, this does not indicate the starting position was equal to 0. Documentation must specify whether the range of motion was active or passive.

12. Answer: 3   Resource: Rothstein (995)

Protective asepsis for respiratory isolation includes a mask. Examples of conditions that may require respiratory isolation include measles, mumps and pertussis.

13. Answer: 4   Resource: Thomas (168)

Athetosis refers to involuntary movements characterized as slow, irregular and twisting. This type of motor disturbance makes it extremely difficult to maintain a static body position.

14. Answer: 2   Resource: Thomas (132)

Wernicke's aphasia refers to an inability to comprehend written or spoken words. As a result of this condition it is inappropriate to provide detailed instructions.

15. Answer: 2   Resource: Guide for Professional Conduct

Determining weightbearing status is the responsibility of the referring physician.

16. Answer: 3   Resource: Pierson (314)

Although it is strongly recommended that healthcare employees receive the hepatitis B vaccine, it is not mandated by OSHA.

17. Answer: 1   Resource: Minor (290)

The parallel bars provide the most stable setting for the client to begin ambulation activities.

18. Answer: 4   Resource: Pierson (193)

A walker with a platform attachment will provide the stability the client requires while avoiding significant pressure on both of the fracture sites.

19. Answer: 2   Resource: Pierson (123)

A sliding board transfer is possible based on the client's upper extremity strength. The transfer will allow the client to maintain a high level of independence.

20. Answer: 4   Resource: Magee (247)

Full extension and supination is the close packed position of the ulnohumeral joint.

21. Answer: 3   Resource: Hoppenfeld (101)

The flexor digitorum profundus is responsible for flexing the distal interphalangeal joint of the four fingers and assisting with flexion of the proximal interphalangeal and metacarpophalangeal joints.

22. Answer: 1   Resource: Magee (534)

The iliotibial band serves as a secondary restraint to the anterior cruciate ligament not the posterior cruciate ligament.

23. Answer: 2   Resource: Bly (63)

Rolling from prone to supine usually occurs in the fifth month, while rolling from supine to prone occurs in the sixth month.

24. Answer: 4   Resource: Campbell (961)

An Individualized Education Plan articulates the goals and objectives of special education services for a given school aged child. The plan is for a one year period.

25. Answer: 2   Resource: Michlovitz (198)

A client report of a slight burning sensation under the soundhead can be due to inadequate coupling, loosening of the crystal or hot spots due to a high beam nonuniformity ratio.

26. Answer: 4   Resource: Irwin (366)

The optimal position for the superior segments of the lower lobes is described as having the client lie on his/her abdomen with two pillows under the hips. The therapist claps over the middle back at the tip of the scapula on either side of the spine.

27. Answer: 4   Resource: Irwin (5)

A phase II cardiac rehabilitation program begins with the completion of a low level treadmill test and ends with a maximal treadmill test.

28. Answer: 3   Resource: Goold (32)

Positioning the client in supine with the legs elevated would be inappropriate first aid management. This position may be warranted in a client with hypovolemic shock.

29. Answer: 2   Resource: Ciccone (35)

The kidneys are the primary site of drug excretion, while the gastrointestinal tract and lungs are secondary sites.

30. Answer: 4   Resource: Kisner (615)

Bilateral straight leg raising is contraindicated for a pregnant woman due to the excessive increase in abdominal pressure and the strain on the low back.

31. Answer: 1   Resource: Michlovitz (140)

Buoyancy makes the body appear to weigh less in water than it does in air and as a result clients tend to move with greater ease when immersed in water.

32. Answer: 1   Resource: Michlovitz (213)

Diathermy is considered a deep heating agent while the remaining options are superficial heating agents.

33. Answer: 1   Resource: Magee (283)

The deformity is most frequently encountered in clients with rheumatoid arthritis or after trauma. It is caused by damage to the central tendinous slip of the extensor hood.

34. Answer: 3   Resource: Brannon (106)

Clients with congestive heart failure may present with breathlessness, weakness, abdominal discomfort and edema in the lower extremities resulting from venous stasis. Since sodium serves to retain water it is often restricted in a client's diet.

35. Answer: 4   Resource: Hilt (345)

Clinical union provides the necessary bony support to terminate external fixation. Callus formation represents the first stage in which bony union occurs, however does not offer adequate support.

36. Answer: 3   Resource: Pauls (74)

Ankylosing spondylitis is a form of rheumatic disease characterized by inflammation of the spine resulting in back pain. Since a client with ankylosing spondylitis often exhibits postural changes such as forward head, increased thoracic kyphosis and loss of lumbar curvature, spinal extension exercises are often a component of a treatment regiment.

37. Answer: 4   Resource: Standards of Practice

It is an appropriate action to request additional physical therapy visits from a referring physician.

38. Answer: 3   Resource: Magee (196)

Full shoulder medial rotation is necessary to reach the perineum.

39. Answer: 3   Resource: Pierson (267)

Any change in color or odor of urine is significant and should therefore be reported and documented.

40. Answer: 4   Resource: Robinson (182)

An orthotic device such as the Milwaukee brace is designed to facilitate improved alignment in the developing spine and therefore should be used until spinal growth ceases.

41. Answer: 2   Resource: Ciccone (329)

Dizziness, shortness of breath and coughing up blood are all symptoms that place a client's safety in immediate jeopardy.

42. Answer: 3   Resource: Kettenbach (125)

Equipment needs and equipment ordered are typically included in the plan section of a S.O.A.P. note.

43. Answer: 2   Resource: Walters (250)

Productivity is a term used to describe the efficiency of a given worker or group of workers. Although measures of quality are often examined concurrently they are not used to determine productivity.

44. Answer: 4   Resource: Magee (2)

The self referred client offers a medical history that presents several significant issues including episodes of dizziness, neck stiffness with pain at night and a family history of cancer. Based on the client's history and the date of the medical examination he should be referred to a physician.

45. Answer: 3   Resource: Brannon (316)

A perceived exertion scale is a subjective scale where clients rate their exercise intensity.

46. Answer: 2   Resource: Goodman (25)

Open-ended questions guide the discussion, but do not restrict information to categories. Closed-ended questions are more impersonal and provide a limited number of response options.

47. Answer: 3   Resource: Standards of Practice

Direct personal contact with the referring physician is necessary to plan an effective care plan.

48. Answer: 4   Resource: Magee (212)

A Bankart lesion is an avulsion of the capsule and glenoid labrum off of the anterior rim of the glenoid resulting from traumatic anterior dislocation of the shoulder. Since the subscapularis is placed on stretch with external rotation this motion is initially limited after surgery.

49. Answer: 3   Resource: Rothstein (17)

According to the Americans with Disabilities Act Accessibility Guidelines the distance necessary for a 180 degree turn using a wheelchair is 60 inches.

50. Answer: 3   Resource: Ellis (162)

All of the listed tasks are reasonable expectations for the client, however moving from sitting to standing would be the most difficult.

51. Answer: 4   Resource: Pierson (293)

Due to the probability associated with incidental contact, the front of the gown below waist level is considered to be non sterile.

52. Answer: 3   Resource: Norkin and White (72)

Stabilization should occur on the distal humerus to prevent shoulder flexion.

53. Answer: 3   Resource: Ellis (15)

A supine position will ensure client safety and allow the therapist full access to the residual limb.

54. Answer: 1   Resource: Pauls (161)

Leaving the residual limb exposed to the air at all times would result in increased edema and a misshapened residual limb.

55. Answer: 4   Resource: Pierson (267)

Positioning of the collection bag on the wheelchair leg rest will allow for it to be below the level of the bladder.

56. Answer: 2   Resource: Minor (290)

The client's balance and strength require the stability provided by the walker.

57. Answer: 4   Resource: O'Sullivan (103)

Ataxia refers to defective muscular coordination with active movement. A gross measures of upper extremity ataxia can be assessed through a finger to nose test.

58. Answer: 2   Resource: Sullivan - Clinical Decision Making (71)

Rhythmic initiation is a particularly effective technique to improve motor control in clients with Parkinson's disease since they often have difficulty initiating movement.

59. Answer: 4   Resource: O'Sullivan (98)

Clients with cerebellar degeneration often exhibit hypotonia, not hypertonia.

60. Answer: 3   Resource: Umphred (247)

Prone over a wedge positioning allows for the facilitation of head and back extension through visual tracking or upper extremity movement occurring during therapeutic play.

61. Answer: 2   Resource: Ratliffe (26)

Head positioning is the stimulus for the symmetrical tonic neck reflex. When the head is flexed, upper extremities flex and lower extremities extend. When the head extends the upper extremities extend and lower extremities flex. The reaction of the extremities would not allow for maintaining a hands and knees position.

62. Answer: 2   Resource: Davis (119)

Inappropriate behavior is unacceptable and should not be tolerated. The therapist needs to make the client aware that her behavior is inappropriate and offensive.

63. Answer: 3   Resource: Guide for Professional Conduct

Scheduling with another therapist will allow the client to be seen two times a week as indicated on the referral and will accommodate the client's schedule.

64. Answer: 4   Resource: Kettenbach (83)

Well written goals contain four distinct elements: audience, behavior, condition and degree.

65. Answer: 1   Resource: Umphred (716)

An articulation at the ankle joint would allow the tibia to advance forward over the fixed foot. This would assist with weight shifting during the sit to stand transfer.

66. Answer: 1   Resource: Brannon (3)

A maximum heart rate increase of 20 beats per minute above resting is considered a safe guideline for a client participating in a phase I program.

67. Answer: 3   Resource: Davis (88)

The response "surgery can be a very frightening thought" is an empathetic response that demonstrates respect for the client's feelings.

68. Answer: 4   Resource: Brannon (206)

Anxiety, tobacco, alcohol and caffeine consumption can all serve to precipitate preventricular contractions. Sodium has not been shown to have any direct correlation.

69. Answer: 1   Resource: Robinson (23)

Phase charge is represented by the area under a single phase waveform. The unit of measure is the coulomb.

70. Answer: 2   Resource: Minor (302)

Guarding should occur with one hand positioned on the client's shoulder and the other on the hip. If a gait belt is used the lower hand should grasp the gait belt with the forearm in a supinated position.

71. Answer: 4   Resource: Pierson (152)

Increased pressure in the popliteal area can lead to skin irritation and circulatory compromise.

72. Answer: 2   Resource: Norkin (320)

The gluteus maximus and the hamstrings function as primary hip extensors. These muscles function in an eccentric fashion when moving from standing to sitting.

73. Answer: 2   Resource: Walter (244)

Quality assurance programs which focus on process explore the methods, actions and operations used to bring about a specific result.

74. Answer: 4   Resource: Standards of Practice

The physician should be informed about the client's lack of progress. The client may be discharged from physical therapy or referred back to the physician.

75. Answer: 2   Resource: Paz (378)

Anemia refers to a reduction in the number of circulating red blood cells. Additional symptoms include vertigo, weakness, headache and general malaise.

76. Answer: 4   Resource: Ciccone (7)

Although over the counter medications contain low doses of their active ingredients, harmful effects can occur.

77. Answer: 1   Resource: Kisner (610)

This position will tend to lessen the effects of uterine compression on abdominal vessels and improve cardiac output by turning the client slightly to the left.

78. Answer: 4   Resource: Kendall (284)

Muscle testing of the middle trapezius should occur with the client in the prone position.

79. Answer: 3   Resource: Ratliffe (197)

A client with spastic diplegia often utilizes mobility strategies such as "bunny hopping" due to the lack of dissociation of the lower extremities from each other as well as the trunk from the pelvis. These activities should be discouraged and the focus should instead be on dissociation and reciprocal movement patterns.

80. Answer: 2   Resource: Tecklin (194)

For thoracic and high level lumbar lesions the parapodium provides the necessary amount of support and is optimal to assist with standing activities. The parallel bars are the most stable assistive device to initiate standing and to utilize during formal gait training.

81. Answer: 1   Resource: Umphred (221)

Premature infants do not have the prolonged intrauterine environment which assists in the development of flexion. There is a high risk for the infant to develop excessive extension and therefore should not be positioned in full extension in the supine position. Positioning should focus on facilitating flexion.

82. Answer: 4   Resource: Michlovitz (272)

Ultraviolet light combined with topical psoralens has proven to be effective in treating psoriasis.

83. Answer: 1   Resource: Robinson (6)

Ampere is the standard unit of measure for current.

84. Answer: 4   Resource: Scott - Promoting Legal Awareness (65)

Although a variety of subjective and objective data are admissible in a court of law, formal documentation is often paramount.

85. Answer: 1   Resource: Pierson (221)

This position affords the therapist with the best opportunity to protect the client in the event of a fall.

86. Answer: 3   Resource: Kisner (639)

Clients with chronic venous insufficiency must wear compression stockings during periods of activity such as ambulation in order to avoid venous stasis and promote return to the heart.

87. Answer: 2   Resource: Post-Stroke Rehabilitation (74)

The client's dependence with ambulation and transfers eliminate home care as a viable option.

88. Answer: 3   Resource: Irwin (360)

Segmental breathing can be an effective treatment technique designed to direct activity toward selected areas of the lung.

89. Answer: 2   Resource: Brannon (260)

A decrease in systolic blood pressure of greater than 10 mmHg or failure of systolic blood pressure to rise with an increase in work load are indications to discontinue a graded exercise test.

90. Answer: 2   Resource: Minor (228)

A sliding transfer with drawer sheet is the only transfer which will allow the client to maintain a position of less than 30 degrees elevation.

91. Answer: 4   Resource: Pierson (293)

Sterile objects that touch each other are still considered sterile.

92. Answer: 4   Resource: Ellis (15)

Encouraging proximal joint flexion can lead to contractures.

93. Answer: 2   Resource: Norkin and White (5)

The frontal plane divides the body into front and back halves. Movements in the frontal plane occur as side to side movements such as abduction or adduction. Rotary motion in the frontal plane occurs around an anterior-posterior axis.

94. Answer: 3   Resource: Sullivan - Clinical Decision Making (64)

Maintained pressure is an effective technique that can be used to increase range of motion by facilitating local muscle relaxation, however it is a passive technique.

95. Answer: 4   Resource: Minor (34)

An irregular pulse should be taken for 60 seconds in order to achieve an accurate measurement.

96. Answer: 2   Resource: Pierson (195)

The parallel bars should be adjusted to provide 15 - 25 degrees of elbow flexion with a client in standing and holding the parallel bars six inches anterior to his/her hips.

97. Answer: 2   Resource: Irwin (364)

Postural drainage to the posterior segments of the upper lobes is performed with the sitting, leaning over a pillow at a 30 degree angle.

98. Answer: 4   Resource: Pierson (150)

Seat width = hip width + 2 inches
Seat depth = posterior buttock to the popliteal space - 2 inches

99. Answer: 4   Resource: Thomas (96)

Anemia is defined as a reduction in the number of circulating red blood cells per cubic millimeter. Symptoms of anemia include pallor of the skin, vertigo and general malaise.

100. Answer: 1   Resource: Buchanan (227)

Heterotopic ossification refers to abnormal bone growth in tissue. Signs and symptoms include decreased range of motion, local swelling and warmth. Heterotopic ossification often occurs in clients following a head injury.

101. Answer: 1   Resource: Pierson (193)

A walker provides more stability than axillary crutches and is more functional than the parallel bars.

102. Answer: 3   Resource: Kettenbach (72)

The problem list should summarize the significant findings of the client as determined by the subjective and objective examination. Since the problem list relates back to the subjective and objective portion of the note each entry should be described in broad terms.

103. Answer: 3   Resource: The Educator's Guide to the ADA (96)

Questions asked during interviews should only relate to the functions associated with a given job and should not probe into an applicant's past medical or social history.

104. Answer: 2   Resource: Pierson (268)

External catheters are applied over the shaft of a penis and are therefore inappropriate for females.

105. Answer: 2   Resource: Pierson (266)

In order to promote optimal fluid flow from an IV when ambulating, a client should grasp the pole so the infusion site is at heart level.

106. Answer: 4   Resource: Pierson (57)

The width of a bladder should be approximately 40% of the circumference of the mid point of the limb. Bladder width for an average size adult is 5-6 inches.

107. Answer: 2   Resource: Kettenbach (8)

Although typewritten entries in the medical record are acceptable, they are not required.

108. Answer: 3   Resource: Code of Ethics

The only viable solution to meet the client's physical need is to allow him to use the bathroom.

109. Answer: 3   Resource: Pierson (109)

A client status post total hip replacement using an anterolateral surgical approach would be most restricted in external rotation. Failure to restrict external rotation may result in hip dislocation or subluxation.

110. Answer: 3   Resource: Pierson (50)

Pulse rate is increased with anxiety or stress.

111. Answer: 3   Resource: Davis (85)

Suggesting the client write down questions for the physician is a practical and realistic option that will assist her in future interactions.

112. Answer: 1   Resource: Brannon (134)

Beta-blockers decrease heart rate and the force associated with myocardial contraction. On an electrocardiogram they may cause sinus bradycardia.

113. Answer: 3   Resource: Michlovitz (99)

Ice massage is an accessible and effective cryotherapeutic agent that is often incorporated into a home exercise program to reduce inflammation.

114. Answer: 4   Resource: Kisner (443)

Many individuals are able to continue to function at high levels despite a variety of ligamentous and meniscal injuries, therefore functional instability provides the most direct support for an anterior cruciate ligament reconstruction.

115. Answer: 3   Resource: Davis (85)

In order to determine if the client's poor attendance in therapy is due to difficulty understanding the scheduling card, the information must be presented in a manner that the client can understand.

116. Answer: 1   Resource: Brannon (3)

Although resting levels of heart rate and blood pressure were not provided, a heart rate of 125 beats/minute and a respiration rate of 32 breaths/minute exceed typical values.

117. Answer: 1   Resource: Clark (339)

TLSOs prevent thoracic flexion and are most commonly prescribed in cases of fracture or compression of the body of the lower thoracic or upper lumbar vertebrae. TLSOs are sometimes referred to as a "Jewett brace."

118. Answer: 4   Resource: Post-Stroke Rehabilitation (232)

The Fugl-Meyer has been proven to have good validity and reliability for assessing motor function and balance in clients with hemiplegia.

119. Answer: 1   Resource: Hoppenfeld (203)

The cuboid is located on the lateral aspect of the foot immediately posterior to the styloid process of the fifth metatarsal.

120. Answer: 3   Resource: Guide for Professional Conduct

The therapist should not alter the client's weightbearing status without prior physician approval.

121. Answer: 4   Resource: Pierson (265)

A nasogastric tube is a plastic tube that enters the body through a nostril and terminates in a client's stomach. As a result the tube is not used for obtaining venous samples.

122. Answer: 2   Resource: Minor (344)

Clients using axillary crutches often lean forward on the crutches to support the body during periods of standing. This activity can lead to damage in the axillary region.

123. Answer: 2   Resource: Norkin and White (104)

Carpometacarpal flexion occurs in a frontal plane around an anterior-posterior axis with the client in the anatomical position.

124. Answer: 1   Resource: Ellis (12)

Frequent prone positioning is important for clients with transfemoral and transtibial amputations, however clients with transfemoral amputations are more susceptible to a hip flexion contracture.

125. Answer: 2   Resource: Paz (334)

Post-polio syndrome is a term used to describe symptoms that occur years after the onset of poliomyelitis. The condition is believed to result as remaining motor units become more dysfunctional. Sensation is typically not affected by post-polio syndrome.

126. Answer: 2   Resource: Paz (334)

Clients with Parkinson's disease often exhibit difficulty initiating movement, rigidity, absence of equilibrium responses and diminished associated reactions.

127. Answer: 2   Resource: Magee (303)

Assembling small bolts, nuts and washers are activities used in a number of assessment measures which examine fine motor coordination such as the Purdue Peg Board Test.

128. Answer: 1   Resource: Rothstein (592)

Approximate blood pressure by age; 10 years old 90/60 mmHg, 30 years old 115/75 mmHg, 50 years old 125/82 mmHg, 70 years old 135/88 mmHg.

129. Answer: 3   Resource: Minor (39)

Age predicted maximum heart rate = 220 - age. Maximum heart rate = 220 - 29 = 191.

130. Answer: 4   Resource: Guide to Physical Therapist
                                                              Practice

The physical therapy aide is a non licensed worker who is trained under the direction of a physical therapist. Aides are involved in client related and non-client related duties, however, would not be responsible for implementing an exercise program.

131. Answer: 2   Resource: Davis (87)

"Try to utilize your own strength to complete the transfer" is a direct statement which should present the client with a clear understanding of the therapist's objective. It also places the client in an active instead of a passive position.

132. Answer: 3   Resource: Magee (539)

Since all clients have different degrees of ligamentous laxity it is essential to establish a baseline with the uninvolved extremity prior to assessing the involved extremity.

133. Answer: 1   Resource: Guide for Professional Conduct

The length of the car ride makes therapy three times a week unrealistic. If reducing the number of therapy visits jeopardizes the outcome of care, it may be appropriate to find therapy services within a more narrow geographic radius.

134. Answer: 1   Resource: O'Sullivan (384)

Clips often provide poor anchors and can cut the skin. Safety pins are also of questionable value, however are not as dangerous as clips.

135. Answer: 1   Resource: Robinson (285)

Conventional TENS utilizes a pulse rate of 50-100 pps, short pulse or phase duration and low intensity to deliver sensory level stimulation.

136. Answer: 4   Resource: Michlovitz (132)

Treatment should be discontinued when there is any sign of heat intolerance. It is important to document the incident in order to alert other possible providers to the client's reaction and to make the incident part of the permanent medical record.

137. Answer: 4   Resource: Sullivan - An Integrated
                                              Approach (89)

The modified plantigrade position requires clients to possess control of equilibrium and proprioceptive reactions. The position offers a small base of support and high center of gravity with weightbearing occurring through the lower extremities.

138. Answer: 4   Resource: Minor (299)

A swing through gait pattern relies on the same principles as a swing to gait pattern, however allows a client to bring the lower extremities beyond the point to which the assistive devices were advanced.

139. Answer: 1   Resource: Haggard (74)

Hands on training sessions provide unique opportunities for the therapist to assess the competence of family members in a structured environment.

140. Answer: 4   Resource: Guide for Professional Conduct

Therapists should never place their personal safety in jeopardy.

141. Answer: 2   Resource: Norkin and White (4)

The sagittal plane divides the body into left and right halves. Motions in the sagittal plane include flexion and extension. Bilateral shoulder flexion would create the largest forward movement and would therefore provide the greatest challenge for the client.

142. Answer: 2   Resource: Hoppenfeld (279)

Shortening of the latissimus dorsi often presents as a limitation of shoulder flexion or abduction due to the muscles origin on the external lip of the iliac crest and its insertion on the intertubercular groove of the humerus.

143. Answer: 2   Resource: Arends (47)

The psychomotor domain is directed toward physical activity. The six categories of objectives in the psychomotor domain according to Bloom's taxonomies are reflex movements, basic fundamental movements, perceptual abilities, physical abilities, skilled movements and non discursive communications.

144. Answer: 3   Resource: Pierson (281)

The first and most appropriate action is to put on gloves. Although direct pressure over the laceration is necessary, a therapist must always protect him/herself first.

145. Answer: 1   Resource: Adkins (146)

Self range of motion of the lower extremity is a realistic goal at the C7 spinal injury level, but not at C5.

146. Answer: 4   Resource: Buchanan (139)

This activity requires the least skill and will provide the client with the opportunity to gain a sense of balance before moving to more difficult activities.

147. Answer: 4   Resource: Guide to Physical Therapist
                                                          Practice (1-10)

A physical therapist assistant can modify a specific intervention procedure when necessitated by a change in client status, however cannot alter an established plan of care.

148. Answer: 4   Resource: Kendall (277)

The upper fibers of the pectoralis major are innervated by the lateral pectoral nerve C5,6,7.

149. Answer: 2   Resource: O'Sullivan (511)

A superficial partial thickness burn involves both the epidermis and a portion of the dermis. Healing typically occurs in approximately three weeks with little or no scarring.

150. Answer: 2   Resource: Currier (52)

Institutional review boards are responsible for assuring the welfare and safety of clients and establishing that ethical, moral and legal standards are not compromised by proposed research activity.

151. Answer: 3   Resource: Edelman (158)

Sensitivity can be calculated by taking the number of individuals the instrument identified as diseased, who were diseased, and dividing by the known prevalence of the condition in the group.

152. Answer: 4   Resource: Pierson (267)

Failure to allow for adequate flow of urine into a collection bag can lead to serious medical complications.

153. Answer: 4   Resource: Pierson (36)

The elbow is not typically in direct contact with a given component of a wheelchair and is therefore not likely to be the site of a pressure ulcer.

154. Answer: 1   Resource: Guide for Professional Conduct

An adolescent with a moderate scoliotic curve should be referred to a physician for further assessment.

155. Answer: 3   Resource: Pierson (149)

Nine inches above the chair seat allows the typical user to sit upright with the shoulders level while bearing weight on the forearms positioned on the armrests.

156. Answer: 3   Resource: O'Sullivan (502)

Clients in the confused-agitated stage have a short attention span and therefore require numerous activities.

157. Answer: 3   Resource: Adkins (186)

Friction surface handrims assist a client without a strong grasp.

158. Answer: 1   Resource: Michlovitz (116)

Hot packs should be stored in water that is approximately 160 degrees Fahrenheit or 71 degrees Celsius.

159. Answer: 3   Resource: Currier (108)

Systematic sampling requires a list of all individuals in a defined population. Members of the population are automatically selected once the first subject has been chosen.

160. Answer: 1   Resource: Kisner (196)

The resting position is a position in which the capsule has the greatest laxity. As a result there is maximal joint traction and joint play.

161. Answer: 2   Resource: Best (262)

Rejecting the null hypothesis at the .01 level indicates the researcher is taking a 1% risk of encountering a Type I error.

162. Answer: 4   Resource: Guide for Professional Conduct

The therapist should not provide additional services when he/she believes the client will no longer benefit from therapy.

163. Answer: 2   Resource: Irwin (342)

It is often necessary to examine upper, middle and lower lobe expansion during quite and deep breathing.

164. Answer: 4   Resource: Paz (630)

Vocational dysfunction is not associated with pressure sores. Other risk factors include diminished sensation, infection, spasticity and disuse atrophy.

165. Answer: 4   Resource: O'Sullivan (525)

Splinting in elbow extension and forearm supination will effectively limit contractures and maximize functional use of the upper extremity.

166. Answer: 1   Resource: Nelson (255)

The process of electromyography involves asking a client to move a particular muscle so that voluntary potentials can be recorded. There should not be any recorded electrical activity in a muscle at rest.

167. Answer: 2   Resource: Hoppenfeld (122)

C7 level: Motor - triceps, wrist flexors, finger extensors
Sensation - middle finger
Reflex - triceps

168. Answer: 4   Resource: Magee (176)

Acromioclavicular dysfunction often results in a painful arc from 120-180 degrees of abduction. A painful arc from 90-120 degrees may be indicative of subacromial bursitis, calcium deposits or tendonitis of the rotator cuff muscles.

169. Answer: 3   Resource: Umphred (734)

Changing the client's environment and staff frequently will yield to greater levels of stress and cognitive dysfunction.

170. Answer: 2   Resource: Norkin - Joint Structure and Function (458)

Cadence is defined as the number of steps taken by a person per unit of time.

171. Answer: 3   Resource: Pauls (654)

Osteoporosis refers to a disease process that results in a reduction of bone mass. Screening by measuring height can provide an inexpensive method to screen for this disease.

172. Answer: 3   Resource: Brannon (317)

Walking at 3 mph, bicycling at 6 mph or playing golf while pulling a bag cart are activities which require 3-4 METs.

173. Answer: 3   Resource: O'Sullivan (418)

A client walking at a comfortable pace with a transfemoral prosthesis requires nearly 50% more oxygen than normal.

174. Answer: 3   Resource: Standards of Practice

It is important to document any delay in the initiation of physical therapy services and to notify the referring physician.

175. Answer: 1   Resource: Kendall (209)

The test for the lateral hamstrings is described with the knee in 50-70 degrees of flexion with the thigh in slight lateral rotation and the leg in slight lateral rotation on the thigh. Pressure should be applied against the leg proximal to the ankle in the direction of knee extension.

176. Answer: 1   Resource: Irwin (348)

Respiratory acidosis is caused by retention of carbon dioxide due to pulmonary insufficiency. Signs and symptoms include dizziness, tingling and syncope.

177. Answer: 3   Resource: Guide for Professional Conduct

The client is likely to be intoxicated if he has consumed six or seven beers. Contacting a member of the family will prevent the possibility of the client attempting to drive.

178. Answer: 2   Resource: Kisner (711)

Reducing the weight to five pounds will allow the client to maintain the integrity of the originally prescribed exercise, while allowing the client to perform the exercise correctly.

179. Answer: 1   Resource: Pierson (311)

A bandage is used to secure underlying dressing and therefore does not come in direct contact with the wound.

180. Answer: 1   Resource: Thomas (503)

A client with moderate dementia can not live independently without assistance and frequent supervision. Without adequate support the clients safety is jeopardized.

181. Answer: 4   Resource: Pauls (329)

Guillain-Barre is an acute polyneuropathy causing rapid, progressive loss of motor function. Although mild sensory loss can be evident, absent sensation is extremely rare.

182. Answer: 2   Resource: Pauls (337)

Multiple sclerosis is a progressive disease of the central nervous system marked by intermittent damage to the myelin sheath. Blurred vision and muscle weakness are common symptoms associated with this condition.

183. Answer: 4   Resource: Michlovitz (233)

Internal or external metal objects are contraindications for shortwave and microwave diathermy.

184. Answer: 1   Resource: Pierson (159)

Removable armrests will assist the client when transferring from wheelchair to bed. Elevating legrests can limit the amount of time the involved leg is in a dependent position.

185. Answer: 1   Resource: Magee (635)

The talar tilt test is performed with the client in supine with the knee flexed to 90 degrees. The foot should be maintained in a neutral position while the foot is moved from side to side into abduction and adduction. A positive test is indicated by excessive adduction.

186. Answer: 4   Resource: O'Sullivan (502)

Clients that are confused-agitated are often over stimulated by busy environments.

187. Answer: 3   Resource: Shumway-Cook (16)

The Motor Control / Task Oriented Approach theorizes that movement is organized around a goal behavior. It also believes that strategies for moving are elicited when a client interacts with the environment during a functional task.

188. Answer: 1   Resource: Kettenbach (125)

The word "will" denotes future tense. This entry is most appropriate in the plan section of a S.O.A.P. note.

189. Answer: 1   Resource: Minor (294)

A rolling walker will provide the client with the necessary stability to ambulate safely. The wheels will allow for a smoother more coordinated gait pattern.

190. Answer: 1   Resource: Minor (308)

When ascending stairs clients should follow the normal flow of traffic. Since the client does not have unilateral weakness it is most appropriate to ascend the stairs on the right. This necessitates holding the canes with the left hand and grasping the handrail with the right.

191. Answer: 4   Resource: Umphred (424)

Decorticate posturing is characterized by abnormal flexor responses in the upper
extremity and extensor responses in the lower extremities. The posture is usually
indicative of a lesion at or above the upper brain stem.

192. Answer: 2   Resource: Ratliffe (27)

The positive support reflex promotes extension of the lower extremities and trunk with
weightbearing through the balls of the feet. This reflex normally integrates at two months
of age.

193. Answer: 1   Resource: Kisner (196)

Grade I or II oscillation or slow intermittent grade I or II sustained joint distraction are
primarily utilized for pain.

194. Answer: 2   Resource: Magee (475)

Anteversion refers to the degree of angulation of the neck of the femur. In adults the
mean is 8-15 degrees. Clients with excessive anteversion often exhibit more than 60
degrees of hip medial rotation and decreased lateral rotation.

195. Answer: 1   Resource: Robinson (340)

Direct current is necessary to ensure a unidirectional flow of ions.

196. Answer: 4   Resource: Campbell (101)

The hip is required to flex during initial swing to allow for proper clearance and
advancement of the limb during gait. Normally, dorsiflexion also occurs. Without the
use of the dorsiflexors the hip flexors need to be strengthened in order to attain proper
clearance.

197. Answer: 3   Resource: Sullivan - An Integrated
                                                  Approach (133)

When resistance is applied against a strong component of a pattern it can result in
irradiation or overflow of impulses to the weaker muscle groups in that pattern.

198. Answer: 3   Resource: Brunnstrom (45)

Stage Four in Brunnstrom's six stages of recovery for hemiplegia consists of a client's
progression to allow for movements performed outside of synergy patterns.

199. Answer: 2   Resource: Sullivan - An Integrated
                                                  Approach (80)

Bridging causes the muscles of the low back and hip extensors to isometricaly contract.
This action promotes hip stability.

200. Answer: 3   Resource: Magee (482)

Clients with tight hip flexors often exhibit an increased lordosis. Shortness of the hip flexors is seen in standing as lumbar lordosis with an anterior pelvic tilt or it can be assessed using the Thomas test.

Bibliography

Adkins H: Spinal Cord Injury, Churchill Livingstone, 1985

Advanced Learning System, The Exeter Consulting Group

American Heritage Dictionary, Dell Publishing Company, 1983

A Guide to Physical Therapist Practice, Volume I: A Description of Patient
     Management, American Physical Therapy Association, 1995

American Red Cross: Emergency Response, The American National Red Cross, 1997

Arends R: Learning to Teach, McGraw-Hill Inc., 1991

Arnheim D: Essentials of Athletic Training, Third Edition, Mosby-Year Book, Inc.,
     1995

Barbe W, Milone M: What We Know About Modality Strengths, Educational
     Leadership, 1981

Berger K: The Developing Person Through The Lifespan, Worth, 1994

Best J, Kahn J: Research in Education, Prentice-Hall, 1986

Bly L: Motor Skill Acquisition in the First Year, Therapy Skill Builders, 1994

Bobath B: Adult Hemiplegia: Evaluation and Treatment, Heinemann Medical Books
     Limited, 1978

Bonwell C, Eison J: Active Learning, Higher Education Reports, 1991

Booher J, Thibodeau G: Athletic Injury Assessment, Times Mirror/Mosby College
     Publishing, 1989

Bootzin R, Acoceila J: Abnormal Psychology, Random House, 1984

Brannon F, Foley M, Starr J, Saul L: Cardiopulmonary Rehabilitation: Basic Theory
     and Application, Second Edition, F.A. Davis, 1998

Brunnstrom S: Movement Therapy in Hemiplegia, Harper and Row Publishers Inc.,
     1970

Buchanan L, Nawoczenski D: Spinal Cord Injury: Concepts and Management
     Approaches, Williams & Wilkins, 1987

Cameron M: Physical Agents in Rehabilitation: From Research to Practice, W.B.
     Saunders Company, 1998

Campbell S, Physical Therapy for Children, Second Edition, W.B. Saunders, 2000

Carpenter M: <u>Core Text of Neuroanatomy</u>, Williams & Wilkins, 1985

Ciccone C: <u>Pharmacolgy in Rehabilitation</u>, Second Edition, F.A. Davis, 1996

Clark C, Bonfiglio M: <u>Orthopaedics: Essentials of Diagnosis and Treatment</u>, Churchill Livingstone, 1994

<u>Code of Ethics</u>, American Physical Therapy Association, 1991

Currier D: <u>Elements of Research in Physical Therapy</u>, Williams & Wilkins, 1984

Curtis K: <u>The Physical Therapist's Guide to Health Care</u>, Slack Incorporated, 1999

Daniels K, Worthingham C: <u>Muscle Testing Techniques of Manual Examination</u>, W.B. Saunders, 1986

Davies P: <u>Steps to Follow</u>, Springer-Verlag, 1985

Davis C: <u>Patient Practitioner Interaction</u>, Third Edition, Slack Inc., 1998

De Domenico G, Wood E: <u>Beard's Massage</u>, W.B. Saunders Company, 1997

Domholdt E: <u>Physical Therapy Research Principles and Application</u>, W.B. Saunders Company, Philadelphia, 1993

Dunn, Beaudry, Klavis: "Survey of Research on Learning Styles", <u>Educational Leadership</u>, 1989

Edelman C, Mandle C: <u>Health Promotion</u>, Mosby, 1990

<u>Educator's Guide to the Americans with Disabilities Act</u>, American Vocational Association, 1993

Ellis P, Mensch G: <u>Physical Therapy Management of Lower Extremity Amputations</u>, Aspen Publishers, 1986

Epler M, Palmar L: <u>Manuscript Draft, Graduate Program in Physical Therapy at Massachusetts General Hospital</u>

<u>Examination Handbook for Physical Therapist and Physical Therapist Assistant</u>, Federation of State Boards of Physical Therapy, 1999

Feder B: <u>The Complete Guide to Taking Tests</u>, Prentice Hall, 1979

Fenlon M, Mueller S: <u>Preparing Students for Standardized Testing</u>, 1977

<u>First Aid in the Work Place</u>, Goold, Prentice Hall, 1995

Garrison S: Physical Medicine and Rehabilitation Basics, J.B. Lippincott Company, 1995

Gifford C, Fluitt J: <u>Test Taking Skills and Test Wiseness</u>, 1978

Giles S: _A Guide to Success: Review for Licensure in Physical Therapy_, Mainely Physical Therapy, 1999

Giles S, Stuart J: _Test Master: Physical Therapist Examination_, Mainely Physical Therapy, 2000

Goldenson R: _Disability and Rehabilitation Handbook_, McGraw Hill, 1978

Goodman C, Snyder T: _Differential Diagnosis in Physical Therapy_, W.B. Saunders Company, 1995

Goold G: _First Aid in the Workplace_, Prentice Hall, 1995

Guide to Physical Therapist Practice, American Physical Therapy Association, 1999

Guide for Professional Conduct, American Physical Therapy Association, 1999

Guyton M: _Textbook of Medical Physiology_, W.B. Saunders Company, 1986

Haggard A: _Handbook of Patient Education_, Aspen Publishers, 1989

Hamill J, Knutzen K: _Biomechanical Basis of Human Movement_, Williams & Wilkins, 1995

Hermann N: _The Creative Brain_, Brain Books, 1990

Hertling D, Kessler R: _Management of Common Musculoskeletal Disorders_, Third Edition, Lippincott, 1996

Hickock R: _Physical Therapy Administration and Management_, Williams & Wilkins, 1982

Hill J: _The Problem-Oriented Approach to Physical Therapy Care_, American Physical Therapy Association, 1987

Hilt N, Cogburn S: _Manual of Orthopedics_, 1980

Hoppenfeld S: _Physical Examination of the Spine and Extremities_, Appleton-Century-Crofts, 1976

Irwin S, Tecklin J: _Cardiopulmonary Physical Therapy_, C.V. Mosby Company, 1995

Kendall F, McCreary E: _Muscle Testing and Function_, Williams & Wilkins, 1993

Kettenbach G: _Writing S.O.A.P. Notes_, Second Edition, F.A. Davis, 1995

Kisner C, Colby L: _Therapeutic Exercise Foundations and Techniques_, F.A. Davis, 1996

Magee D: _Orthopedic Physical Assessment_, W.B. Saunders Company, 1997

Mahler D: _American College of Sports Medicine Guidelines for Exercise Testing and Prescription_, Lippincott Williams & Wilkins, 1995

Matthews J: Practice Issues in Physical Therapy, Slack Incorporated, 1989

McConnell J: Understanding Human Behavior, CBS College Publishing, 1983

Michlovitv S: Thermal Agents in Rehabilitation, Third Edition, F.A. Davis, 1996

Miller-Keane: Encyclopedia & Dictionary of Medicine, Sixth Edition, Nursing & Allied Health, W.B. Saunders, 1997

Minor M, Minor SD: Patient Care Skills, Fourth Edition, Appleton & Lange, 1999

Moore K: Clinically Oriented Anatomy, Williams & Wilkins, 1985

National Safety Council First Aid & CPR, Jones and Bartlett Publishers, 1997

Nelson, Barbara, Dunn, Griggs, Primavera, Fitzpatrick, Bacilious, Miller: "Effects of Learning Style Intervention on College Students' Retention and Achievement", Journal of College Student Development, 1993

Nelson R, Currier DP: Clinical Electrotherapy, Appleton-Century-Crofts, 1987

Nixon V: Spinal Cord Injury-A Guide to Functional Outcomes in Physical Therapy Management, Aspen Publishers, 1985

Norkin C, White D: Measurement of Joint Motion: A Guide to Goniometry, Edition Two, F.A. Davis, 1995

Norkin C, Levangie P: Joint Structure & Function, F.A. Davis, 1992

Ornstein, Thompson: The Amazing Brain, Houghton-Mifflin Company, 1984

O'Sullivan S, Schmitz T: Physical Rehabilitation: Assessment and Treatment, F.A. Davis, 1994

Pagliarulo M: Introduction to Physical Therapy, Mosby-Year Book, Inc., 1996

Pauls T, Reed K: Quick Reference to Physical Therapy, Aspen Publishers, 1996

Payton, Hueter, McDonald: "Learning Style Preferences of Physical Therapy Students in the United States", Physical Therapy, 1979

Paz J, Panik M: Acute Care Handbook for Physical Therapists, Butterworth Heinemann, 1997

Phillips A: Test Taking Skills: Incorporating Them into the Curriculum, 1983

Pierson F: Principles and Techniques of Patient Care, Second Edition, W.B. Saunders Company, 1994

Post Stroke Rehabilitation, U. S. Department of Health and Human Services, 1995

Purtilo R: Health Professional and Patient Interaction, Fifth Edition, W.B. Saunders Company, 1996

Raffel M, Raffel N: The United States Health System, Delmar Publishers Inc., 1994

Ratliffe K: Clinical Pediatric Physical Therapy: A Guide for the Physical Therapy Team, Mosby Company, 1998

Richardson A: "Verbalizer-Visualizer: A Cognitive Style Dimension," Journal of Mental Imagery, 1977

Robinson A, Snyder-Mackler L: Clinical Electrophysiology, Williams & Wilkins, 1995

Rothstein J, Roy S, Wolf S: The Rehabilitation Specialists' Handbook, F.A. Davis, 1998

Roy S, Irvin R: Sports Medicine: Prevention, Evaluation, Management and Rehabilitation, Prentice-Hall, 1983

Scott R: Health Care Malpractice, Slack Incorporated, 1990

Scott R: Professional Ethics: A Guide for Rehabilitation Professionals, Mosby Inc., 1998

Scott R: Promoting Legal Awareness in Physical and Occupational Therapy, Mosby 1997

Shumway-Cook A, Woollacott M: Motor Control: Theory and Applications, Williams & Wilkins, 1995

Soderburg G: Kinesiology: Application to Pathological Motion, Williams & Wilkins, 1986

Snyder-Mackler L, Robinson A: Clinical Electrophysiology: Electrotherapy and Electrophysiologic Testing, Williams & Wilkins, 1989

Spinal Cord Injury Concepts and Management Approaches, Williams & Wilkins, 1987

Standards of Practice for Physical Therapy and the Accompanying Criteria, American Physical Therapy Association, 1999

Sullivan S, Markos P, Minor M: An Integrated Approach to Therapeutic Exercise, Reston Publishing Company, 1982

Sullivan P, Markos P: Clinical Decision Making in Therapeutic Exercise, Appleton & Lange, 1995

Tecklin J: Pediatric Physical Therapy, Edition Three, Lippincott Williams & Wilkins, 1999

Thomas C: Taber's Cyclopedic Medical Dictionary, Edition 18, F.A. Davis, 1997

Trofino R: Nursing Care of the Burn Injured Patient, F.A. Davis, 1991.

Umphred D: Neurological Rehabilitation, Third Edition, Mosby Company, 1995

Wade, Carole, Travis: <u>Psychology</u>, Harper Collins College Publishers, 1993

Wadsworth C: <u>Manual Examination and Treatment of the Spine and Extremities</u>, Williams & Wilkins, 1988

Walter J: <u>Physical Therapy Management</u>, Mosby, 1993

Waxman S, deGroot J: <u>Correlative Neuroanatomy</u>, Appleton & Lange, 1995

Zadai C: <u>Clinics in Physical Therapy - Pulmonary Management in Physical Therapy</u>, Churchill Livingstone, 1992

Appendix

Activity Log

	Day One	Day Two	Day Three
8:00			
9:00			
10:00			
11:00			
12:00			
1:00			
2:00			
3:00			
4:00			
5:00			
6:00			
7:00			
8:00			
9:00			

Time Management Diagnostic Sheet

	Day One	Day Two	Day Three	Total
CLASS				
STUDY				
INDIVIDUAL TIME				
SOCIAL TIME				
EXERCISE				
WORK				
SLEEP				
NAP				
NIGHT				
SPECIAL APPOINTMENTS				

Relaxation Exercise

Periodically as indicated by your learning style, use the sample relaxation exercise to relieve your body of unwanted anxiety and stress. Each of the steps should be completed in a slow and somewhat exaggerated manner.

1. Take a deep breath and expire slowly.

2. Close your eyes tightly for 10 seconds and slowly open them.

3. Lift your shoulders towards your ears.

4. Make a tight fist and flex your elbows.

5. Squeeze your buttocks tightly and hold for 3 seconds.

6. Extend your knees and plantarflex your ankles.

7. Close your eyes tightly for 10 seconds and slowly open them.

8. Take a deep breath and expire slowly.

Resource List

American Physical Therapy Association
1111 North Fairfax Street
Alexandria, Virginia 22314
(800) 999-2782
Website: www.apta.org
Fax on demand: (800) 399-2782

Federation of State Boards of Physical Therapy
2231 Crystal Drive, Suite 500
Arlington, Virginia 22202
(703) 299-3100
Website: www.fsbpt.org

Mainely Physical Therapy
P.O. Box 7242
Scarborough, Maine 04070-7242
(207) 885-0304
Website: www.ptexams.com
Fax: (207) 883-8377
email: ptexams@cybertours.com

Professional Examination Service
Interstate Reporting Service
111 8th Avenue, Suite 526
New York, NY 10011-5290
(212) 367-4365

Physical Therapy State Licensing Agencies

Alabama

Alabama Board of Physical Therapy
100 North Union Street, Suite 627
Montgomery, AL 36130-5040
(334) 242-4064

Alaska

State Physical Therapy Board
Division of Occupational Licensing
P.O. Box 110806
Department of Commerce
Juneau, AK 99801-0806
(907) 465-2551

Arizona

State Board of Physical Therapy Examiners
1400 W. Washington, Suite 230
Phoenix, AZ 85007
(602) 542-3095

Arkansas

State Board of Physical Therapy
9 Shackleford Plaza, Suite 1
900 South Shackleford
Little Rock, AR 72211
(501) 228-7100

California

PT Examining Committee
1418 Howe Avenue, Suite 16
Sacramento, CA 95825
(916) 263-2550

Colorado

Division of Registrations
1560 Broadway, Suite 670
Denver, CO 80202
(303) 894-2440

Connecticut

Department ofPublic Health
Physical Therapy Licensure
410 Capitol Avenue, MS 13ADJ
P.O. Box 340308
Hartford, CT 06134-0308
(860) 509-7566

Deleware

Deleware Board of PT
861 Silver Lake Boulevard
Cannon Bldg., Suite 203
Dover, DE 19904-2467
(302) 739-4522

District of Columbia

D.C. Board of Physical Therapy
Dept. of Consumer and Regulatory Affairs
Professional Licensing Administration
614 H Street, NW, Room 923
Washington, DC 20001
(202) 727-7454

Florida

Dept. of Professional Regulation
2020 Capitol Circle, SE
BIN# CO5
Tallahassee, FL 32399-0789
(850) 488-0595

Georgia

State Board of Physical Therapy
State Examining Boards
166 Pryor Street, SW
Atlanta, GA 30303
(404) 656-3921

Hawaii

Dept. of Commerce & Consumer Affairs
Professional Licensing Division
Board of Physical Therapy
1010 Richards Street, P.O. Box 3469
Honolulu, HI 96813
(808) 586-3000

Idaho

Idaho Board of Medicine
280 North 8th Street, Suite 202
P.O. Box 83720
Boise, ID 83720-0058
(208) 334-2822

Indiana

Health Professions Bureau
402 West Washington Street, Room 041
Indianapolis, IN 46204
(317) 232-2960

Kansas

Kansas State Board of Healing Arts
235 S.W. Topeka Boulevard
Topeka, KS 66603
(785) 296-7413

Louisiana

State Board of PT Examiners
2014 W. Pinhook, #701
Lafayette, LA 70508
(318) 262-1043

Maryland

Board of Physical Therapy Examiners
4201 Patterson Avenue, Suite 318
Baltimore, MD 21215-2299
(410) 764-4752

Michigan

Health Licensing Division
P.O. Box 30018
Lansing, MI 48909
(517) 241-9289

Illinois

Department of Professional Regulation
320 West Washington, 3rd Floor
Springfield, IL 62786
(217) 782-8556

Iowa

Department of Public Health
Bureau of Professional Licensure
Board of Physical Therapy Examiners
4th Floor, Lucas Building
Des Moines, IA 50319-0075
(515) 281-4401

Kentucky

State Board of Physical Therapy
9110 Leesgate Road, Suite 6
Louisville, KY 40222-5159
(502) 595-4687

Maine

Board of Examiners in Physical Therapy
Dept. of Professional Regulation
State House Station #35
Augusta, ME 04333
(207) 624-8600

Massachusetts

Board of Allied Health
100 Cambridge Street, Room 1513
Boston, MA 02202
(617) 727-3071

Minnesota

Board of Medical Practice
Physical Therapy Advisory Council
University Park Plaza
2829 University Avenue SE, Suite 400
St. Paul, MN 55414-3246
(612) 617-2130

Mississippi

Mississippi State Department of Health
Professional Licensure Division
P.O. Box 1700
Jackson, MS 39215-1700
(601) 987-4153

Montana

Department of Commerce
Division of Public Safety
Board of Physical Therapy Examiners
P.O. Box 200513
111 North Jackson
Helena, MT 59620-0513
(406) 444-3728

Nevada

State Board of Physical Therapy Examiners
P.O. Box 81467
Las Vegas, NV 89180-1467
(702) 876-5535

New Jersey

New Jersey State Board of PT
124 Halsey Street, 6th Floor
P.O. Box 45014
Newark, NJ 07101
(201) 504-6455

New York

State Board for Physical Therapy
State Education Department
Cultural Education Center, Room 3019
Albany, NY 12230
(518) 474-6374

North Dakota

North Dakota State Examining
Committee for Physical Therapists
P.O. Box 69
Grafton, ND 58237
(701) 352-0125

Missouri

Missouri Board of Healing Arts
P.O. Box 4
Jefferson City, MO 65102
(573) 751-0144

Nebraska

Department of Health and Human Services
Physical Therapy
301 Centennial Mall South
Lincoln, NE 68509-5007
(402) 471-2115

New Hampshire

Board of Registration in Medicine
2 Industrial Park Drive
Concord, NH 03301
(603) 271-1203

New Mexico

New Mexico PT Licensing Board
P.O. Box 25101
725 St. Michael's Drive
Santa Fe, NM 87504
(505) 476-7130

North Carolina

Board of Physical Therapy Examiners
18 West Colony Place, #120
Durham, NC 27705
(919) 490-6393

Ohio

Ohio Physical Therapy Board
77 South High Street, 16th Floor
Columbus, OH 43266-0317
(614) 466-3774

Oklahoma

Oklahoma State Board of Medicine
P.O. Box 18256
5104 North Francis, Suite C
Oklahoma City, OK 73154-0256
(405) 848-6841

Pennsylvania

State Board of Physical Therapy
P.O. Box 2649
Harrisburg, PA 17105-2649
(717) 783-7134

Rhode Island

Rhode Island Department of Health
Division of Professional Regulation
3 Capitol Hill
104 Cannon Building
Providence, RI 02908-5097
(401) 277-2827

South Dakota

Board of Medical and Osteopathic Examiners
1323 South Minnesota Avenue
Sioux Falls, SD 57105
(605) 334-8343

Texas

Board of Physical Therapy Examiners
333 Guadalupe, Suite 2-510
Austin, TX 78701-3942
(512) 305-6900

Vermont

Office of Professional Regulation
Office of the Secretary of State
Licensing and Registration Division
109 State Street
Montpeiler, VT 05609-1106
(802) 828-2390

Oregon

Physical Therapy Licensing Board
800 NE Oregon Street, Suite 407
Portland, OR 97232
(503) 731-4047

Puerto Rico

Office of Regulation & Certification
Profession of Health
Call Box 10200
Santurce, PR 00908-0200
(809) 725-8161 ext. 209

South Carolina

Board of Physical Therapy Examiners
110 Centerview Drive
P.O. Box 11329
Columbia, SC 29211-1329
(803) 896-4655

Tennessee

Tennessee Board of O.T./P.T Examiners
1st Floor Cordell Hull Building
425 5th Avenue North
Nashville, TN 37247-1010
(615) 532-5136

Utah

Division of Professional Licensing
160 East 300 South
P.O. Box 146741
Salt Lake City, UT 84114-6741
(801) 530-6621

Virgin Islands

Board of Physical Therapy Examiners
Department of Health
48 Sugar Estate
St. Thomas, VI 00802
(809) 774-0117

Virginia

Department of Health Professions
Board of Medicine
1601 Rolling Hills Drive
Richmond, VA 23229-5005
(804) 662-9073

West Virginia

West Virginia Board of Physical Therapy
JW Davis Government Building
153 West Main Street, Suite 103
Clarksburg, WV 26301
(304) 745-4161

Wyoming

State Board of Physical Therapy
First Bank Plaza
2020 Carey Ave, Suite 201
Cheyenne, WY 82002
(307) 777-3507

Washington

Department of Health
1300 SE Quince Street
P.O. Box 47868
Olympia, WA 98504-7868
(360) 753-3132

Wisconsin

Dept. of Regulation and Licensing
Medical Examining Board
P.O. Box 8935
Madison, WI 53708
(608) 266-2811

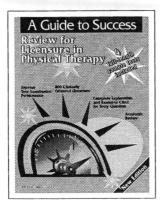

A Guide to Success
Review for Licensure in Physical Therapy

A Guide to Success consists of two major sections. The first is a review of a physical therapy academic curriculum and is designed to serve as a review and a resource.

The second section is a compilation of four sample examinations designed to be reflective of the current Physical Therapist Examination.

■ Contents

• Comprehensive academic review provides rapid access to essential examination information

• Explanation and resource cited for all examination questions

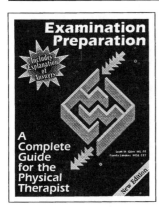

Examination Preparation
A Complete Guide for the Physical Therapist

Examination Preparation is designed to allow candidates to take an active role in their preparation for the Physical Therapist Examination. Sample exercises and assessment activities provide candidates with individual feedback on their current performance.

The text will allow candidates to:
• Learn valuable test-taking strategies
• Explore in detail the content outline of the Physical Therapist Examination

• Develop a comprehensive study plan
• Answer hundreds of sample questions with explanations and resources cited

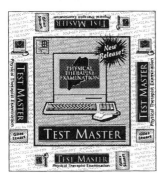

Test Master
Physical Therapist Examination

TEST MASTER allows candidates to experience computer based testing and at the same time gather valuable information on their examination performance.

This innovative software program operates on Microsoft Windows '98 or '95 and requires a 386/25MHz, 8 MB RAM and 6 MB disk space.

■ Contents

• Two complete sample examinations designed to the exact specifications of the current Physical Therapist Examination

• Explanation and resource cited for all examination questions
• Detailed performance analysis according to area of Clinical Practice and the Content Outline

▪ ORDERING INFORMATION ▪

TITLE	QUANTITY	PRICE EACH	TOTAL
A Guide to Success – PT		39.95	
Examination Preparation – PT		33.95	
Test Master – PT (Diskettes)		35.95	
		Shipping Charges	$4.00
		ORDER TOTAL	

Method of Payment

☐ I've enclosed check # _____ payable to Mainely Physical Therapy

☐ Please charge to:

☐ Mastercard ☐ Visa Exp. Date __ __/__ __

☐ Card No._____-_____-_____-_____

☐ Signature _____
REQUIRED TO PROCESS ORDER

Ship to:

Name _____

Address_____

City_____ State____ Zip_____

PT School _____

Phone # (____) _____

▪ ORDERING OPTIONS ▪

Mail
Mainely Physical Therapy
P.O. Box 7242
Scarborough, ME 04070-7242

when you order the
Save $15!
"Ultimate Review"

Internet
http://ptexams.com

Phone
(207) 885-0304

THIS BUNDLE INCLUDES:
■ A Guide to Success
■ Examination Preparation
■ Test Master
Cost $94.85
Actual Retail Value $109.85

Fax
(207) 883-8377

BUNDLE	QUANTITY	PRICE EACH	TOTAL
"Ultimate Review" – PT		94.85	
		Shipping Charges	$4.00
		ORDER TOTAL	